Orthopaedics
in
Primary Care

Edited by

Andrew J Carr, ChM, FRCS
Consultant Orthopaedic Surgeon,
Nuffield Orthopaedic Centre,
Oxford

Anthony Harnden, MRCP, MRCGP, DCH
General practitioner,
Norland House Surgery,
Wheatley,
Oxfordshire

D1424131

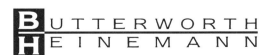

BUTTERWORTH
HEINEMANN

Butterworth-Heinemann
Linacre House, Jordan Hill, Oxford OX2 8DP
225 Wildwood Avenue, Woburn, MA 01801-2041
A division of Reed Educational and Professional Publishing Ltd

A member of the Reed Elsevier plc group

OXFORD   BOSTON   JOHANNESBURG
MELBOURNE   NEW DELHI   SINGAPORE

First published 1997
Reprinted 1998 (twice)

British Library Cataloguing in Publication Data
Orthopaedics in primary care
  1. Orthopaedics
  I. Carr, Andrew J. II. Harnden, Anthony
  617.3

ISBN 0 7506 2219 9

Library of Congress Cataloguing in Publication Data
Orthopaedics in primary care / edited by Andrew J. Carr, Anthony
  Harnden.
  p. cm.
  Includes bibliographical references and index.
  ISBN 0 7506 2219 9
  1. Orthopaedics 2. Primary care (Medicine) I. Carr, A. (Andrew)
  II. Harnden, Anthony
  [DNLM: 1. Orthopaedics. 2. Primary Health Care. WE 168 076278]
  RD732.0778
  616.7-dc21   96-37668
                                                            CIP

Composition by Scribe Design, Gillingham, Kent
Printed and bound in Great Britain by MPG Books Ltd, Bodmin, Cornwall

Contents

Preface

The accurate diagnosis and appropriate management of orthopaedic musculoskeletal problems presents a considerable challenge to general practitioners. Recent data from the National Morbidity Study (1990–91) shows that 10% of all clinical contact in general practice is for a musculoskeletal problem. Morbidity in the community is even greater and with an ageing population will continue to rise. Most orthopaedic problems are managed successfully within general practice – those referred on to secondary care are in the minority. Orthopaedic clinicians practising in secondary care are privy to only a small fraction of orthopaedic problems in the community and will inevitably have a skewed impression of relative frequency and distribution of these problems. The purpose of this book, drawing on the expertise of both orthopaedic surgeons and general practitioners, was to develop a text that describes common and important orthopaedic complaints in the context of a primary care setting. It is not a text written by orthopaedic surgeons for general practitioners but a collaborative exercise between general practitioners and orthopaedic surgeons. The book is intended to be an information source for busy general practitioners. It brings ideas of better orthopaedic practice in primary care that will help improve clinical effectiveness.

The process used for the development of each chapter was important. Authors were asked to produce a draft outline which was sent to a group of five or more Oxford general practitioners, prior to an evening meeting. (Twenty-eight general practitioners participated in total.) The composition of the groups varied with each chapter. The meetings stimulated discussions following which the chapters were revised – new sections added, some expanded, contracted and deleted – in order to give a balanced text reflecting orthopaedic problems presenting in primary care. The general practitioners found the small group discussions together with the demonstration of joint injection techniques educationally extremely valuable. These educational methods will form a cornerstone for future orthopaedic postgraduate courses for general practitioners in Oxford.

The chapters have common themes. Each text provides a thorough, but not comprehensive, description of orthopaedic problems a general practitioner might encounter during the course of their work, paying particular attention both to those problems occurring frequently and to those which might only be encountered rarely but present significant diagnostic and management issues. During the evening meetings groups highlighted important messages, which are summarized at the beginning of each chapter. Authors produced a set of case histories, the answers they felt correct are standardized for each chapter. They are the authors' views of best management and are intended to provoke debate. Where appropriate the chapters contain illustrations of normal ranges of joint movement, examples of joint injection techniques and radiological findings. Tables display age-related pathology and postoperative expectations for common operations.

Although this book is primarily directed towards general practitioners, it is hoped that medical students, orthopaedic surgeons in training and other allied professional groups will find it useful. We feel it is essential, with ever increasing models of shared care and a blurring of the margins between primary and secondary care, that both consultant and general practitioner have an understanding of the type and pattern of orthopaedic problems presenting within each sector.

The following general practitioners, without whose enthusiasm and constructive criticism this book would not have been possible are acknowledged: Martin Agass, Pat Alquist, Julie Anderson, Neil Bryson, Ken Burch, Andy Chivers, Anthony Clarke, Ian Eastwood, Andrew Farmer, Nigel Gilmour, Richard Green, Richard Harrington, Tim Huins, John Humphreys, Peter Isaac, Claudia Jones, Duncan Keeley, Tim Lancaster, Veronica McKay, Jane Mortensen, Ben Parker, David Parker, Simon Plint, Michael Robertson, Peter Rose, Gill Scott, Judy Shakespeare, Simon Street, Tim Wilson and Ken Wiliamson.

Anthony Harnden
Andrew Carr

Contributors

Michael K.D. Benson FRCS Consultant Orthopaedic Surgeon, Nuffield Orthopaedic Centre, Oxford, UK

Simon Bowman PhD, MRCP Consultant Rheumatologist, Birmingham, UK

Peter D. Burge FRCS Consultant Orthopaedic Surgeon, Nuffield Orthopaedic Centre, Oxford, UK

Andrew J. Carr ChM, FRCS Consultant Orthopaedic Surgeon, Nuffield Orthopaedic Centre, Oxford, UK

Paul H. Cooke ChM, FRCS Consultant Orthopaedic Surgeon, Nuffield Orthopaedic Centre, Oxford, UK

Anthony Harnden MRCP, MRCGP, DCH General Practitioner, Norland House Surgery, Wheatley, Oxfordshire

Richard de Steiger FRACS Consultant Orthopaedic Surgeon, Royal Melbourne Hospital, Melbourne, Australia

Christopher A. Dodd FRCS Consultant Orthopaedic Surgeon, Nuffield Orthopaedic Centre, Oxford, UK

Jeremy C.T. Fairbank MD. FRCS Consultant Orthopaedic Surgeon, Nuffield Orthopaedic Centre, Oxford, UK

Jane Moser MSc, MCSP Senior Physiotherapist, Nuffield Orthopaedic Centre, Oxford, UK

John R. Williams MA, FRCS ARC Clinical Research Fellow, Nuffield Orthopaedic Centre, Oxford, UK

James Wilson-MacDonald ChM, FRCS Consultant Orthopaedic Surgeon, Nuffield Orthopaedic Centre, Oxford, UK

Acknowledgements

The figures in Chapter 11 are based on illustrations taken from 'Physiotherapy: General Exercises' by PhysioTools. PhysioTools and PhysioTools Compatible Collections are used to produce personal patient handouts on a PC running Windows. More information is available on the internet at www.physiotools.com.

tel.   +358 208 301 303
fax: +358 207 301 303
e-mail: info@physiotools.com

1
Shoulder

Andrew J. Carr

- Shoulder pain is the next commonest skeletal complaint after back pain to present to GPs.
- A short history and examination will differentiate pathology in the glenohumeral joint from pathology in the subacromial space.
- In primary care the posterior and lateral approaches are easier when injecting steroid into the subacromial bursa.
- Two episodes of shoulder dislocation are an indication for surgical stabilization.

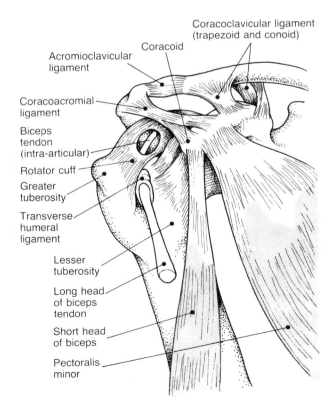

Coracoclavicular ligament
(trapezoid and conoid)

Coracoid

Acromioclavicular ligament

Coracoacromial ligament

Biceps tendon (intra-articular)

Rotator cuff

Greater tuberosity

Transverse humeral ligament

Lesser tuberosity

Long head of biceps tendon

Short head of biceps

Pectoralis minor

Fig. 1.1 *Some of the major ligamentous and musculotendinous attachments about the shoulder joint*

Presenting symptoms

Assessment of the presenting symptoms should differentiate between the three main complaints of patients with shoulder problems. These are **pain, stiffness** and **instability**. Attempts should be made to determine how these symptoms affect working activities, activities of daily living and sporting activities. Pain may be present only on activity (usually above-head activity) but can be present at rest or at night.

Pain and stiffness

1 **is it from the glenohumeral joint?**
    if so pain present day and night
            global restriction of movement including rotation with elbow at side
    then analgesics, NSAIDs, then steroid injections (into joint), then refer (physiotherapy only if predominant problem is stiffness).
2 **is it from the subacromial space?**
    if so pain worse on certain movements
            movements restricted in flexion and abduction
            rotation with elbow at side preserved
    then analgesics, NSAIDs, physiotherapy, then steroid injections into subacromial space, then refer.

Table 1.1 Common causes of shoulder pain in different age groups

	Cause		
Age group	*Intra-articular*	*Periarticular*	*Referred*
Childhood (2–10 years)	Instability	Osteochondromas	
Adolescence (10–18 years)	Instability		
Early adulthood (18–30 years)	Instability Acromioclavicular joint sprain	Calcific tendonitis Impingement	Cervical
Adulthood (30–50 years)	Osteochondritis Osteoarthritis Frozen shoulder Inflammatory arthritis	Calcific tendonitis Impingment Rotator cuff tear Bicipital tendonitis	Cervical
Old age (>50 years)	Osteochondritis Osteoarthritis Frozen shoulder Inflammatory arthritis	Impingment Rotator cuff tear	Cervical

Physical examination

Inspect

Physical examination should begin with an inspection of the shoulder, particularly looking for areas of swelling or muscle wasting.

Palpate

Palpation can often be useful in determining areas of particular tenderness, such as the subacromial region and the greater tuberosity of the humerus or the acromioclavicular joint.

Move

Assess the range of movement in abduction, flexion and external rotation with the elbow at the side. These movements can be expressed in degrees. Internal rotation is best assessed and expressed by examining how far behind the back the patient can get their hand.

An assessment should be made of power or strength in addition to grading strength of abduction and elevation, it is important to assess strength of internal and external rotation, with the elbow tucked into the side.

Table 1.2 Normal range of movement: shoulder

Flexion	0–170 degrees
Abduction	0–170 degrees
External rotation	0–60 degrees
Internal rotation	Hand to upper lumbar spine

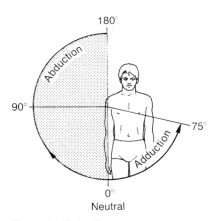

Fig. 1.2 *Abduction*

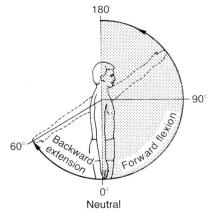

Fig. 1.3 *Flexion*

3

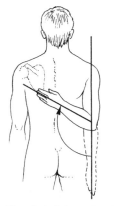

Fig. 1.4 *Internal rotation*

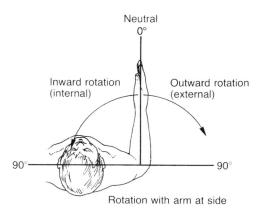

Fig. 1.5 *External rotation*

Pathology in other sites

Examination of the shoulder should always include assessment of the neurology of the upper limb and also assessment of the cervical spine and chest.

Common shoulder problems

Frozen shoulder

This is a common pathology occurring principally in the middle aged and elderly. It often has no precipitating cause, but it may be associated with trauma, cervical spine pathology, diabetes and other metabolic diseases. The characteristic feature of frozen shoulder is a global restriction of movement. Symptoms are probably due to some form of inflammatory process within the capsule of the shoulder joint. The condition tends to be self-limiting, usually lasting no more than 18–36 months.

Physiotherapy often aggravates symptoms in the painful inflammatory phase, but may help when the main problem is stiffness. In particularly symptomatic cases intra-articular injection of lidocaine, and an anti-inflammatory agent is often beneficial. Should symptoms persist in a severe form for more than 3–6 months, then referral for a shoulder opinion is indicated. Arthroscopy and manipulation may help in resistant cases.

In this age group important differential diagnoses are infection and metastatic disease. Impingement symptoms and glenohumeral osteoarthritis can sometimes present with a frozen shoulder picture.

Subacromial impingement (painful arc)

This is a common cause of shoulder symptoms and tends to affect people from age 30 onwards. It is characterized by pain on movement in the shoulder which is worse in particular positions where the greater tuberosity of the humerus impinges against the anterior part of the acromion and the coraco-acromial ligament. It sometimes, but not always, produces a painful arc picture. The symptoms may be bilateral.

Plain radiographs of the shoulder sometimes show evidence of beaking of the acromion and bony changes on the humerus. Initial treatment should be by a series of stretching and strengthening exercises. Local anaesthetic and anti-inflammatory injections into the subacromial region through an anterior or posterior approach may also be beneficial. Should symptoms persist for more than 3–6 months and be resistant to treatment with physiotherapy and injections, then referral is appropriate. These symptoms are sometimes associated with rotator cuff tendon rupture. Subacromial impingement can be treated surgically with arthroscopic decompression.

Rotator cuff tears

Rotator cuff failure is usually degenerative and begins with the supraspinatus tendon and may go on to include the infraspinatus tendon and subscapularis tendon. Symptoms are often similar to those of subacromial impingement, with pain maximal in certain positions of shoulder movement. This is often when the arm is lifted overhead and may prevent any significant overhead activity. Rotator cuff weakness may also be evident on examination and it is particularly important to assess internal and external rotation. Rotator cuff rupture is commonest in the age group 40–60.

Treatment should begin with a series of stretching and strengthening exercises, followed by injections into the subacromial region if physiotherapy fails to show any benefit. Should symptoms persist, particularly pain, then referral is appropriate.

Rotator cuff rupture can be successfully treated surgically with acromioplasty and repair of the rotator cuff tendon tear. Sometimes secondary arthritis occurs in the shoulder joint.

Acromioclavicular joint arthritis

This may present in the age group 40 onwards and sometimes follows earlier trauma to the joint. The pain is often well localized and the joint is usually tender. Treatment with local anaesthetic and steroid injections is often successful. Should symptoms persist, then surgical excision of the outer end of the clavicle may be an appropriate solution.

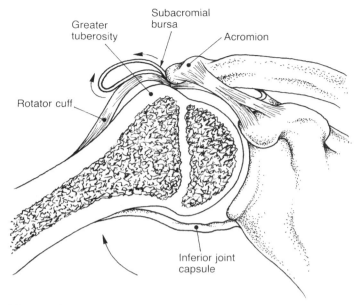

Greater
tuberosity

Subacromial
bursa

Acromion

Rotator cuff

Inferior joint
capsule

Fig. 1.6 *Demonstrating the mechanism of impingement of the rotator cuff and subacromial bursa between the humeral head and overlying coracoacromial arch*

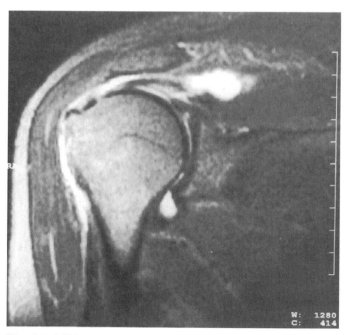

Fig. 1.7 *MRI showing a rotator cuff tear*

Glenohumeral arthritis

Glenohumeral osteoarthritis is less common than arthritis affecting the hip and knee joints. It produces limitations of movement and pain, often occurring at rest and at night. Treatment of early disease with physiotherapy, NSAIDs and steroid injections may be appropriate, but if these fail a referral for consideration of total joint replacement should be made.

Bicipital tendonitis

This is an uncommon condition which causes inflammation of the long head of biceps. It is characterized by tenderness located at the anterior part of the shoulder and in the bicipital groove of the humerus. Physiotherapy may be beneficial and occasionally local anaesthetic and steroid injections produce improvement of symptoms. Surgery is very rarely indicated.

Calcifying tendonitis

Calcifying tendonitis is characterized by deposition of calcium deposits within the rotator cuff muscles, usually the supraspinatus. The symptoms are similar to those of subacromial impingement, with pain and discomfort in certain positions. Treatment should be with physiotherapy to improve the range of movement, followed by local anaesthetic

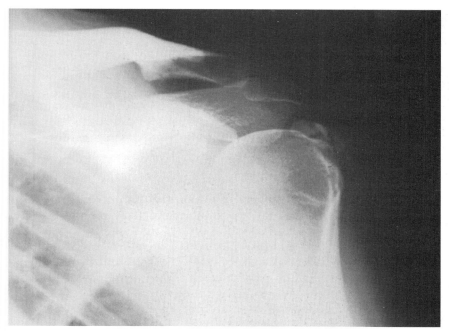

Fig. 1.8 *X-ray of the shoulder showing calcification of the supraspinatus tendon*

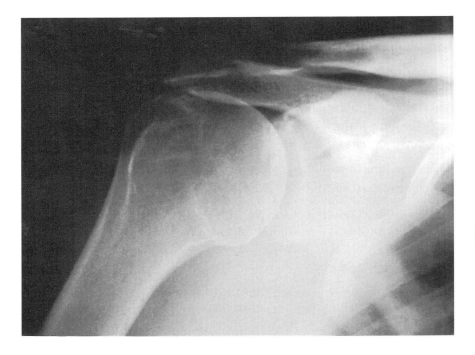

Fig. 1.9 *Radiograph showing subacromial impingement*

and steroid injections. The age group is usual slightly younger than those presenting with rotator cuff tendon ruptures.

Treatment with these conservative methods is usually successful, but occasionally surgery is necessary to excise the calcific deposit and perform an acromioplasty. The surgery can be performed arthroscopically.

Recurrent anterior dislocation

This group of patients is usually young, in their late teens, twenties or early thirties. There is usually a good history of trauma to the shoulder, producing either dislocation or subluxation of the joint. If the capsule on the anterior part of the shoulder fails to heal, then the shoulder is unstable and liable to recurrent subluxation or dislocation. Symptoms are often intermittent, but the patient is very wary of performing certain activities and often has to give up sporting activity. The best treatment for this condition is surgical with stabilization of the shoulder joint using some form of soft tissue operation. Two to three episodes of dislocation or subluxation are usually an indication for surgery.

Multidirectional instability

This condition is much rarer than traumatic anterior dislocation of the shoulder and is associated with a congenitally lax capsule. There is often no good history of trauma and there is a tendency for the shoulder to dislocate in a number of directions. The mainstay of treatment in this condition is physiotherapy and rehabilitation. Referral for advice about appropriate physiotherapy programmes should be done early. Surgery is only rarely indicated and has a much lower success rate than treatment of anterior dislocations.

Acromioclavicular joint dislocation

This usually presents in young people following sporting trauma or a fall from a motorbike or a horse. There is often a visible deformity of the joint on examination. Treatment is with rehabilitation and physiotherapy. Should the dislocation be painful and resistant to this treatment, then referral for consideration of surgical reconstruction should be made. The majority of people are managed satisfactorily with conservative means.

Humeral fractures

Fractures of the proximal humerus in childhood usually involve the neck of the humerus and are invariably treated conservatively. The prognosis is good. In adulthood fractures are often of the neck of the humerus or of the greater tuberosity, sometimes internal fixation is required. In the elderly, particularly where bone is osteoporotic, then the humerus may fracture into three or four fragments. Surgical treatment is sometimes necessary. The prognosis should be guarded, pain and stiffness often occur.

Case histories

1

A 62-year-old has had a painful shoulder for 4 years. The pain has been getting gradually worse. It is most noticeable at night. He notices crepitus whenever he moves his shoulder.

Simple analgesics	1
NSAIDs	1
Rest	1
Physiotherapy	0

Splints/support/bandages	0
Aspiration	0
Steroid injection	0
Blood test	0
X-ray	1
Routine referral	0
Urgent referral	0
Emergency referral	1
None of these	0

Surgeon's view: Osteoarthritis is likely – an X-ray should be performed. NSAIDs may help the pain. If pain persists referral to a shoulder clinic is indicated.

2

A 24-year-old man sustained an anterior dislocation of his right shoulder 8 months ago when playing rugby and has subsequently had four further painful anterior dislocations, initially while playing sport and, on the most recent occasion, in bed. All of these dislocations required sedation for relocation of the joint.

Simple analgesics	1
NSAIDs	0
Rest	0
Physiotherapy	0
Splints/support/bandages	0
Aspiration	0
Steroid injection	0
Blood test	0
X-ray	0
Routine referral	1
Urgent referral	0
Emergency referral	0
None of these	0

Surgeon's view: This is traumatic unidirectional instability of the shoulder and the best treatment is surgical stabilization of the shoulder. The patient should be referred to a surgeon.

3

A 28-year-old man who was skiing fell onto his outstretched right arm sustaining an injury to the right shoulder; he says it felt like the shoulder came out of joint. Since then he has had problems playing sports, with a feeling of instability of the shoulder. He has had no true dislocation and has not sought any specialist advice about it.

Simple analgesics	1
NSAIDs	0
Rest	0
Physiotherapy	1
Splints/support/bandages	0
Aspiration	0
Steroid injection	0
Blood test	0
X-ray	0
Routine referral	1
Urgent referral	0
Emergency referral	0
None of these	0

Surgeon's view: The history is one of recurrent subluxation of the shoulder. Physiotherapy may help. If physiotherapy fails, referral to a shoulder clinic is indicated.

4

A 39-year-old woman presents with gradual onset of pain and discomfort around the left shoulder, made worse on overhead activity and when she reaches behind her back or to brush her hair.

Simple analgesics	1
NSAIDs	1
Rest	0
Physiotherapy	1
Splints/support/bandages	0
Aspiration	0
Steroid injection	1
Blood test	0
X-ray	0
Routine referral	0
Urgent referral	0
Emergency referral	0
None of these	0

Surgeon's view: This history is suggestive of inflammation in the subacromial space, sometimes known as painful arc or impingement syndrome. Treat with analgesic and anti-inflammatory medication and then with physiotherapy in the initial stages. If these treatments fail, she should have an X-ray. A steroid injection into the subacromial space may also be tried.

5

A 48-year-old man with 3 years of pain and discomfort from his right shoulder made worse on movement, particularly on overhead activity. He has noticed some weakness of the shoulder. He has failed to respond to medication and physiotherapy. Two steroid injections produced relief of symptoms for 2–3 weeks only.

Simple analgesics	1
NSAIDs	0
Rest	1
Physiotherapy	0
Splints/support/bandages	0
Aspiration	0
Steroid injection	0
Blood test	0
X-ray	0
Routine referral	1
Urgent referral	0
Emergency referral	0
None of these	0

Surgeon's view: These symptoms suggest subacromial pain. The history of weakness indicates possible damage to the rotator cuff. Referral to a shoulder clinic is advised.

6

A 62-year-old woman with pain from her right shoulder day and night. Made worse by activity and associated with marked stiffness.

Simple analgesics	1
NSAIDs	1
Rest	1
Physiotherapy	0
Splints/support/bandages	0
Aspiration	0
Steroid injection	0
Blood test	0
X-ray	1
Routine referral	1
Urgent referral	0
Emergency referral	0
None of these	0

Surgeon's view: These symptoms suggest either frozen shoulder (adhesive capsulitis) or osteoarthritis of the glenohumeral joint or very rarely a secondary tumour. Treatment is with analgesic and anti-inflammatory medication in the first instance. An X-ray should exclude osteoarthritis or tumour. Should symptoms persist despite these treatments, referral to a shoulder clinic is indicated.

7

A 23-year-old jockey fell from a horse 4 months ago landing on the point of his shoulder, since when he has noticed a prominent bump at the outer end of his clavicle, which is painful and preventing him from performing his work.

Simple analgesics	1
NSAIDs	0
Rest	1
Physiotherapy	1
Splints/support/bandages	0
Aspiration	0
Steroid injection	0
Blood test	0
X-ray	0
Routine referral	0
Urgent referral	0
Emergency referral	0
None of these	0

Surgeon's view: This history suggests disruption of the acromioclavicular joint. In the majority of instances, non-surgical treatment with pain killers in the initial stages and then mobilization is indicated. Should the dislocation continue to be painful after a period of 3–6 months, then referral to a surgical clinic for consideration of reconstruction of the joint is indicated. An X-ray should be performed.

8

A 54-year-old woman who developed gradual onset of moderate pain in the right shoulder with marked restriction of movement in all directions. The pain is worse on attempted movement.

Simple analgesics	1
NSAIDs	1
Rest	1
Physiotherapy	0
Splints/support/bandages	0
Aspiration	0
Steroid injection	1

Blood test	0
X-ray	0
Routine referral	0
Urgent referral	0
Emergency referral	0
None of these	0

Surgeon's view: Symptoms suggest a moderately severe frozen shoulder (adhesive capsulitis). Initial treatment is with analgesic and non-steroidal anti-inflammatory medication. If symptoms fail to settle an X-ray should be performed to exclude osteoarthritis. Steroid injection may also be tried.

9

A 32-year-old presents with a 48-hour history of acute pain, swelling and stiffness over the shoulder. Erythema is noted on the anterior part of the shoulder.

Simple analgesics	1
NSAIDs	0
Rest	0
Physiotherapy	0
Splints/support/bandages	0
Aspiration	0
Steroid injection	1
Blood test	0
X-ray	0
Routine referral	0
Urgent referral	0
Emergency referral	1
None of these	−1

Surgeon's view: Septic arthritis is a likely diagnosis. Emergency referral to hospital is indicated.

10

A 68-year-old man presents with a painless lump suddenly appearing on the anterior aspect of his right upper arm after gardening. He has a full range of shoulder movement.

Simple analgesics	0
NSAIDs	0
Rest	0
Physiotherapy	0

Splints/support/bandages	0
Aspiration	0
Steroid injection	0
Blood test	0
X-ray	0
Routine referral	0
Urgent referral	0
Emergency referral	0
None of these	0

Surgeon's view: History suggests painless rupture of the long head of the biceps. Surgical treatment is not indicated for this condition unless associated with pain from rotator cuff rupture, when surgical repair should be performed.

Lateral injection into the subacromial bursa

Indication

For impingement syndrome, rotator cuff tears and calcific tendonitis.

Technique

Find the anterolateral corner of the acromion (this lies above the bulge of the humeral head) and aim to pass an 18-gauge needle under the acromion and above the humerus.

Usually use 2–5 ml of a combination of **either** 50 mg hydrocortisone acetate, **or** 20 mg triamcinalone, **or** 40 mg methylprednisolone with 1% lidocaine.

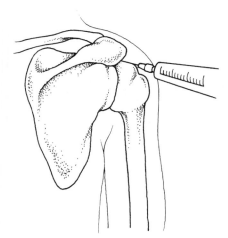

Fig. 1.10 *Lateral approach to the subacromial bursa*

Frequency

Every 4–6 weeks. If there is no benefit after two or three injections, then consider alternative treatment or referral.

Structures at risk

Injection directly onto bone or periosteum is exquisitely painful, so try and avoid it. Also avoid injecting under pressure into tendon as there is a theoretical risk of causing tendon damage.

Posterior injection into the subacromial bursa

Indication

For impingement syndrome, rotator cuff tears and calcific tendonitis.

Technique

Injections in the presence of a joint effusion are relatively easy. However, in adhesive capsulitis or osteoarthritis then injection can be difficult. The posterior approach to the joint is generally more successful and safer.

The entry point is 1 cm distal and medial to the posterior corner of the acromion.

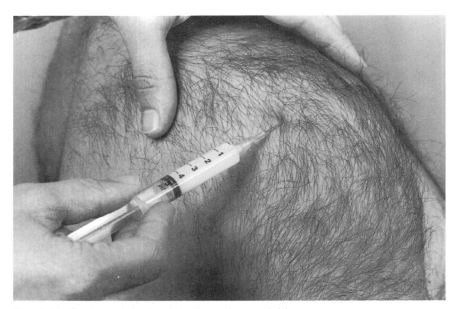

Fig. 1.11 *Posterior injection into the subacromial bursa*

Pass the needle up under the acromion to the full depth of an 18-gauge needle.

Usually use 2–5 ml of a combination of **either** 50 mg hydrocortisone acetate, **or** 20 mg triamcinalone, **or** 40 mg methylprednisolone with 1% lidocaine.

Structures at risk

Injection directly onto bone or periosteum is exquisitely painful, so try and avoid it.

Posterior injection into the glenohumeral joint

Indication

For arthritis or adhesive capsulitis.

Technique

The entry point is 1 cm distal and medial to the posterior corner of the acromion. Head towards the coracoid to the full depth of an 18-gauge needle.

Usually use 2–5 ml of a combination of **either** 50 mg hydrocortisone acetate, **or** 20 mg triamcinalone, **or** 40 mg methylprednisolone with 1% lidocaine.

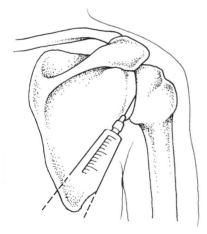

Fig. 1.12 *Injection of the glenohumeral joint: posterior approach*

17

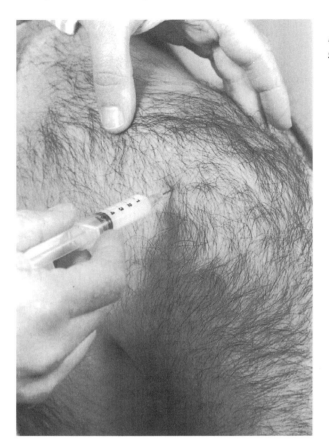

Fig. 1.13 *Posterior injection into the glenohumeral joint*

Structures at risk

Injection directly onto bone or periosteum is exquisitely painful, so try and avoid it.

Further reading

Kelly, I. (ed.) (1993) *The Practice of Shoulder Surgery*. Butterworth–Heinemann, Oxford.

Rockwood, C.A. and Matsen, F.A. (eds) (1990) *The Shoulder*. W.B. Saunders, Philadelphia.

2

Elbow John R. Williams

- A pulled elbow in a child may be treated effectively in primary care without hospital referral.
- Steroid injections for tennis elbow may be repeated for a period of up to 6 months.
- The majority of patients with ulnar nerve entrapment require referral for surgery.

Presenting symptoms

The elbow joint plays an important role, along with the shoulder and wrist joint, in enabling the arm to place the hand in space. Any discussion of the function and pathology of the elbow must include its interaction with the shoulder, wrist and distal radio-ulnar (DRUJ) joints. Pain and stiffness in the elbow joint can restrict many of the activities of daily living such as eating and personal hygiene.

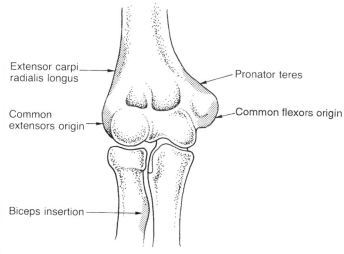

Fig. 2.1 *Muscle insertions around the elbow: anterior view*

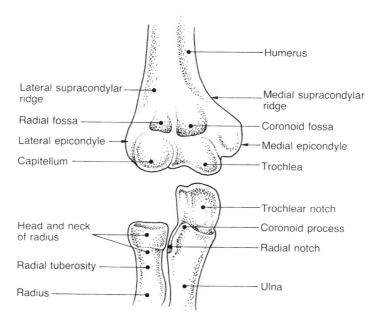

Fig. 2.2 *The bones of the elbow region*

Assessment of elbow symptoms should distinguish between the three main sites of pathology. These are intra-articular damage and/or loose bodies, periarticular soft tissue injury and ulnar nerve lesions at the elbow.

Pain

Insight into the diagnosis is often obtained from the nature of the pain; whether it is constant and present at night or if it is related to particular movements or activities. The latter is particularly the case in sports-related injury. The location of the pain can frequently be helpful. Pain from the lateral joint compartment runs up and down the lateral aspect of the arm and forearm. It must be differentiated from shoulder or cervical root irritation that may radiate down to the elbow or beyond. Medial pain is more commonly associated with medial epicondylitis (golfer's elbow), ulnar nerve entrapment or arthritis.

Physical examination

When examining the elbow it is important to also consider the neck, shoulder, wrist and DRUJ.

Inspect

Inspection of the limb and joint will reveal muscle wasting, gross deformity, soft tissue swelling and the presence of an effusion. Deformity is best displayed with the elbow in the extended position where the normal carrying angle is 10–15 degrees of valgus. Deformities here are commonly caused by intra-articular pathology or growth disturbance following childhood fracture.

Palpate

Palpation of the elbow region should include all four aspects. Laterally one can examine the supracondylar ridge and lateral epicondyle, the lateral joint margins and radial head. The radial head can be fully examined around its edge by rotation of the forearm. Medially the medial epicondyle is felt and behind this the ulnar nerve can be rolled. The origin of the flexor-pronator group of muscles can be palpated. Examination posteriorly should include the olecranon, its bursa and the triceps tendon. Anteriorly the most important structure is the biceps tendon and its insertions.

Move

Movements of the elbow joint occur around two axes. First, flexion and extension from 0 to 140 degrees and secondly rotation around the forearm axis. The normal range of rotation is 75 degrees of pronation and 85 degrees of supination (with the shoulder fixed to prevent abduction or adduction). Loss of terminal passive extension or rotation is an important early indicator of intra-articular pathology. Any loss of range of movement (ROM) should be assessed for firm or soft end points.

The stability of the medial and lateral collateral ligaments can be tested. The medial ligament is test by exerting a valgus force on the forearm with the elbow flexed to 15 degrees to relax the anterior capsule. Similarly, the lateral ligament is tested by a varus stress in the same position of flexion.

Table 2.1 Normal range of movement: elbow

Flexion	0–150 degrees
Pronation	0–80 degrees
Supination	0–80 degrees

Locking

This is relatively uncommon in primary care; however, it has different causes in different age groups. The locking is usually loss of extension

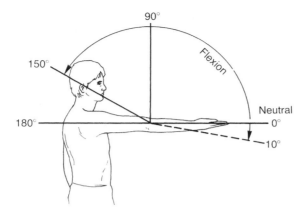

Fig. 2.3 *Flexion and extension*

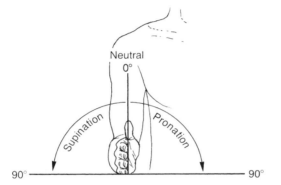

Fig. 2.4 *Pronation and supination*

and occurs intermittently. In young adults it is usually caused by a single loose body following intra-articular trauma or occasionally osteochondritis dissecans. In older patients it is due to osteoarthritis and occasionally synovial chondromatosis.

Common elbow problems

Children

The majority of conditions around the child's elbow are traumatic in origin. A number of congenital disorders affect the elbow, but these are rare. Both cerebral palsy and haemophilia may occasionally be seen affecting the elbow.

Pulled elbow

One traumatic elbow condition which may occasionally present to general practitioners is the pulled elbow or nursemaids elbow. This is usually caused by swinging the child around by the extended arms (or other similar action causing axial forces along the extended arm) and results in the radial head slipping under the edge of the annular ligament. (It rarely has any sinister connotations with non-accidental injury.) The child is commonly between 6 months and 3 years old and accompanied by the distraught adult involved. The child's elbow is painful and he or she will not allow movement from the pronated and flexed position. The treatment is to screw the radial head back through the annular ligament into its normal position by quickly supinating the forearm with axial and valgus strain while in the flexed position. The relocation is often accompanied by a click or pop and immediate relief of pain. Immobilization is rarely required afterwards.

Adults

Overuse conditions

Tennis elbow

This group of conditions which may be acute or chronic commonly present to the medical practitioner. The patient is usually in the 30–55-year-age group. The condition is more accurately known as lateral epicondylitis. Although tennis elbow may be seen in tennis players, this is not exclusively so. It is common in other sports players and occupations that involve repetitive forearm activities (including typing). The pain is localized to the lateral side of the elbow around the origin of extensor group of muscles. Most cases are unilateral, however 10–20% of cases may be bilateral. Those cases that are non-occupational and are caused by one particular, and isolated activity, such as clipping the hedge, usually resolve without any treatment other than reassurance and analgesia if needed.

Tennis elbow often responds to non-operative management if treated in the first few months, but this is less likely to succeed if the problem is of several years' duration. The mainstays of this treatment are rest, pain relief, splintage and injection of the affected area. Rest involves activity modification to avoid excess abuse of the area and may be aided by equipment adjustment, such as racket handle size, and alteration of training regime or correction of position during work. For pain relief NSAIDs are effective. Various arm braces have been used; however, the smaller ones rarely stay in the correct position and the more substantial and effective ones are often unacceptable to the patient. Physiotherapy is not specifically beneficial. If these methods fail a simple injection of local anaesthetic and steroid is indicated. Superficial injection should be avoided, as not only is it not effective but also it may cause skin atrophy changes. Injections may be carried out at 6-weekly to two-monthly intervals. However, if this regularity is required for more than 6 months then other treatments should be sought. Regular injections every 4–6 months, provided that they are placed deeply, are reasonable.

If all these methods fail referral for consideration of surgery should be undertaken. Following surgery the arm should not be immobilized for more than one week. Then gentle strengthening exercises can begin with a planned return to sport or activity at a mild level at 6 weeks.

Golfer's elbow

This is medial epicondylitis occurring in the common flexor origin, and is analogous to tennis elbow occurring on the medial side. Treatment is similar, with the exception that injections must avoid the ulnar nerve lying behind the medial epicondyle. Golfer's elbow may be confused with nerve symptoms from entrapment at the neck, elbow or wrist.

Rheumatoid arthritis

The elbow is frequently affected in rheumatoid arthritis. The rheumatoid elbow should never be viewed in isolation without reference to the shoulder, wrist and hand.

As well as the joint being affected by the destructive arthritis, there may also be rheumatoid nodules and involvement of the olecranon bursa. The proliferative synovium can compromise the function of the nerves at the elbow. Up to 50% of patients with rheumatoid arthritis may develop elbow problems, the majority of which will follow a slow, chronic path.

Rest, splintage and physiotherapy are frequently helpful. The use of analgesics, non-steroidal anti-inflammatories, corticosteroid injections and disease-modifying drugs may be required.

Osteoarthritis

Elbow osteoarthritis is far less common than that of the hip or knee. The majority is secondary to trauma. There are increasing numbers of patients in their forties and fifties presenting with post-traumatic arthritis of the elbow.

These patients present with pain in the joint, often on the lateral side, specifically with activity and at night. There is tenderness around the radial head and along the edge of the ulnar-humeral articulation. There is often a subtle decrease in range of movement, particularly passive terminal extension. Intermittent locking of the joint with pain suggests the development of intra-articular loose bodies. Radiographs are invariably diagnostic.

Initial treatment is symptomatic with analgesics and exercises, followed by joint injection if required. Surgical intervention using arthroscopic techniques allows visualization of the articular surfaces, washout, removal of small loose bodies and limited debridement. Good results are reported after open debridement. Total joint replacement is an option in these patients; however, in patients with high demands on their elbows the success rates are less encouraging than in the rheumatoid patient.

Post-traumatic contracture

This problem is not infrequently encountered following trauma. In the acute situation it should be tackled immediately with physiotherapy and splintage. If these fail and the contracture causes a functional problem then anterior capsulotomy, either arthroscopically or open, may be advocated.

Olecranon bursitis

This may be either traumatic, infective or inflammatory. It is commonly seen in primary care and on most occasions does not require treatment.

Traumatic bursitis may follow a single injury or be due to repeated insult: student's or miner's elbow. Differentiating between septic and inflammatory bursitis can be difficult. A history of fever, marked tenderness and overlying cellulitis would favour an infective cause. A full blood count and aspiration will help in the diagnosis when doubt exists. Radiographs are only helpful in diagnosing an olecranon spur. Septic bursae will require aspiration or surgical drainage, combined with rest, elevation and antibiotic therapy.

Non-septic bursae can usually be treated by symptomatic means and prevention of rubbing. Many practitioners achieve satisfactory results in small and moderate bursae by aspiration and injection of steroids, followed by compression. If the bursa becomes a chronic problem excision can be undertaken. This is often an extensive procedure.

Ulnar nerve entrapment

The most common site of ulnar nerve entrapment is in the cubital tunnel behind the medial epicondyle. This presents as pain down the medial side of the forearm into the ulnar digits. Pain may also extend proximally on the medial side of the arm. The pain is a dull gnawing ache with associated paraesthesia. Sensory changes can be detected in the ulnar digits with reduced two point discrimination and later motor weakness, often initially seen in the first dorsal interosseous muscle. Referral to a specialist is appropriate. The majority of patients will require surgery following electrophysiological confirmation of the site of the lesion.

Case Histories

1

A 47-year-old female typist presents with pain centred over the lateral epicondyle and radiating down the forearm. This is made worse by her work. On examination she had tenderness around the lateral epicondyle and the pain was reproduced by resisting forearm pronation and wrist extension.

Simple analgesia	1
NSAIDs	1
Rest	1
Physiotherapy	0
Splint/support/bandage	0
Aspiration	0
Steroid injection	1
Blood test(s)	0
X-ray	0
Routine referral	0
Urgent referral	0
Emergency referral	0
None of these	0

Surgeon's view: This is tennis elbow. A steroid injection is the best treatment. Physiotherapy is of little help nor is splintage. Modification of position whilst typing may prevent recurrence. Routine referral if injections fail to help.

2

A 24-year-old man who plays cricket at a very good amateur level as a fast bowler complains that he has pain around the medial side of his elbow and that he cannot bowl as well. The pain came on 3 weeks ago and is not present at night. On examination there is no swelling but he is slightly tender in front of the medial epicondyle. Imposing a valgus stress on the elbow reveals asymmetry between the two sides.

Simple analgesia	0
NSAIDs	0
Rest	1
Physiotherapy	1
Splint/support/bandage	1
Aspiration	0
Steroid injection	1
Blood test(s)	0

X-ray	0
Routine referral	1
Urgent referral	0
Emergency referral	0
None of these	0

Surgeon's view: This man has ruptured his medial collateral ligament of the elbow. He has an unstable elbow and will not be able to bowl at his previous level. If he wishes to do this then a surgical reconstruction is advocated.

3

A 54-year-old bricklayer complains that his dominant elbow is painful. This is mainly on the lateral side. It is made worse by his work and occasionally wakes him at night. He has occasional locking of the joint. On examination he has a trace of an effusion within the joint, there was a scar posteriorly where he had some surgery as a child following a fall. The elbow is in 10 degrees more valgus than the other and passive extension is limited at 15 degrees. There is tenderness around the radial head.

Simple analgesia	1
NSAIDs	1
Rest	0
Physiotherapy	0
Splint/support/bandage	0
Aspiration	0
Steroid injection	1
Blood test(s)	0
X-ray	1
Routine referral	1
Urgent referral	0
Emergency referral	0
None of these	0

Surgeon's view: This is a case of post-traumatic osteoarthritis. Like all arthritic conditions the initial treatment is symptomatic. If he fails to respond then routine referral for possible arthroscopy and debridement may be helpful.

4

A 43-year-old carpenter presents with pain on the medial side of his dominant, right forearm. This radiates into the ulnar two fingers at up to the mid part of the medial side of his arm. The discomfort is accompanied by paraesthesia in the little finger. On examination there is tenderness behind the medial epicondyle which reproduces his symptoms. He has some wasting of the first web space.

Simple analgesia	0
NSAIDs	0
Rest	0
Physiotherapy	0
Splint/support/bandage	0
Aspiration	0
Steroid injection	0
Blood test(s)	0
X-ray	0
Routine referral	0
Urgent referral	1
Emergency referral	0
None of these	0

Surgeon's view: This man has a well-developed ulnar nerve palsy which is most probably at the elbow. In view of his muscle wasting he should be referred urgently for consideration of ulnar nerve release and possible anterior transfer.

5

A 22-month-old child is brought to your surgery by his mother. The child will not move his elbow which he holds across his chest. His mother and aunt were swinging him up some steps between them when his arm started hurting. The child is tearful but you elicit that the arm is tender over the radial head and he does not want you to move it.

Simple analgesia	1
NSAIDs	0
Rest	0
Physiotherapy	0
Splint/support/bandage	0
Aspiration	0
Steroid injection	0
Blood test(s)	0
X-ray	0
Routine referral	0
Urgent referral	0
Emergency referral	1
None of these	0

Surgeon's view: The child has a pulled elbow. Reduction can be achieved by the method described.

6

A 55-year-old lady with rheumatoid arthritis complains that her elbows are becoming slowly worse and that she now has difficulty getting out of the chair. She has had previous wrist fusions. Her shoulder movements are fair but her left elbow is swollen and has a restricted range of movement, the right one is less affected.

Simple analgesia	1
NSAIDs	1
Rest	1
Physiotherapy	1
Splint/support/bandage	1
Aspiration	0
Steroid injection	1
Blood test(s)	0
X-ray	0
Routine referral	1
Urgent referral	0
Emergency referral	0
None of these	0

Surgeon's view: This lady's rheumatoid disease is, predictably, affecting her elbows. One must consider her shoulder and wrist joints at the same time. Initial treatment is medical. However, routine referral for consideration of surgery should be made if no improvement is forthcoming.

Medial injection of the elbow

Indications

For golfer's elbow.

Technique

Palpate the point of the medial epicondyle and feel the fleshy substance of the flexor muscles just anterior. The most tender area is often over the periosteum just anterior to the medial epicondyle. However, the pathology appears to be in the muscle and you should aim to inject into the flesh of the flexor muscle to the depth of 1 cm.

Usually use 2 ml of a combination of **either** 10–25 mg hydrocortisone acetate, **or** 5–10 mg triamcinalone, **or** 10–20 mg methylprednisolone with 1% lidocaine.

Frequency

Every 4–6 weeks. If there is no benefit after two to three injections then consider alternative treatment or referral.

Structures at risk

Injection directly onto bone or periosteum is exquisitely painful, so try and avoid it. Also avoid injecting under pressure into tendon as there is a theoretical risk of causing tendon damage.

Try and avoid injecting subcutaneously over the medial epicondyle, as this may be painful and is more likely to cause trophic skin changes.

The ulnar nerve lies just posterior to the medial epicondyle.

Lateral injection of the elbow

Indications

For tennis elbow.

Technique

Palpate the point of the lateral epicondyle and feel the fleshy substance of the extensor muscles just anterior. The most tender area is often over the periosteum just anterior to the lateral epicondyle. However, the pathology appears to be in the muscle and you should aim to inject into the flesh of the extensor muscle to the depth of 1 cm.

Usually use 2 ml of a combination of **either** 10–25 mg hydrocortisone acetate, **or** 5–10 mg triamcinalone, **or** 10–20 mg methylprednisolone with 1% lidocaine.

Frequency

Every 4–6 weeks. If there is no benefit after two to three injections then consider alternative treatment or referral.

Structures at risk

Injection directly onto bone or periosteum is exquisitely painful, so try and avoid it. Also avoid injecting under pressure into tendon as there is a theoretical risk of causing tendon damage.

Try and avoid injecting subcutaneously posterior to the lateral epicondyle, as this may be painful and is more likely to cause trophic skin changes.

The radial nerve lies about 2 cm anterior and medial to the lateral epicondyle.

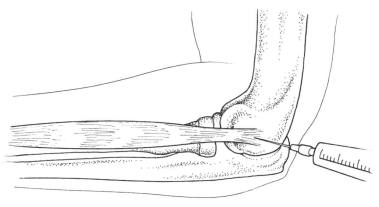

Fig. 2.5 *lateral injection of the elbow*

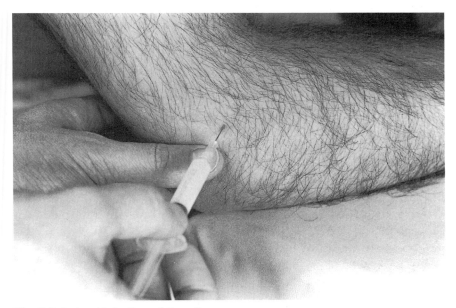

Fig. 2.6 *Lateral injection of the elbow*

Further reading

Barry, M. and Jenner J. R. (1995). ABC of rheumatology. Pain in neck, shoulder and arm. *Br. Med. J.*, **310**; 183.

Morrey, B. F. (1993). *The Elbow and its Disorders*. W.B. Saunders, Philadelphia.

Nicholson, D. A. and Driscoll P. A. (1993). ABC of emergency radiology. The elbow. *Br. Med. J.*, **307**; 1058.

3

Hand and wrist _____ Peter D. Burge

- Seventy per cent of trigger fingers are asymptomatic 1 year after a single injection of steroid.
- The majority of ganglions of the hand and wrist may be successfully managed in primary care.
- Painful hand infections require prompt referral and surgical drainage.
- Dupuytren's disease without contracture is not an indication for referral.

Presenting symptoms

The presentation of hand and wrist problems is very variable. It may include symptoms of pain and restriction of movement, but may also involve neurological symptoms or more specific problems such as those encountered in trigger finger. The hand is also particularly prone to traumatic problems and to infections. It is important to be aware of acute pain and swelling as possible hallmarks of a hand infection; such problems require urgent treatment.

Physical examination

Inspect

Inspection of the hand may reveal evidence of swelling or deformity. Ganglia are the most common cause of swelling in the hand and wrist and usually occur on the posterior surface of the wrist. Deformities of the hand may be due to local problems such as a fascial contracture. However, they may also be due to more proximal neurological disorders.

Palpation

Feeling the hand and wrist may provide clues regarding the location of pain and tenderness. It may also reveal swellings of underlying tissues as may be encountered in trigger finger. Palpation should also include a careful neurological examination.

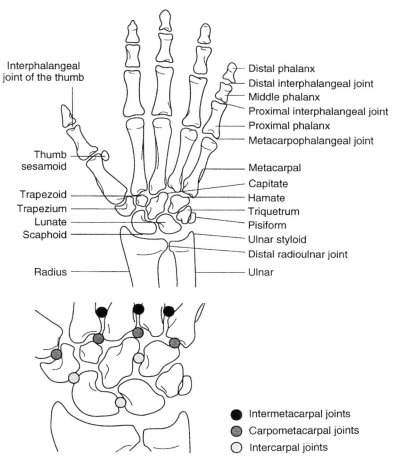

Interphalangeal joint of the thumb

Distal phalanx
Distal interphalangeal joint
Middle phalanx
Proximal interphalangeal joint
Proximal phalanx
Metacarpophalangeal joint

Thumb sesamoid

Metacarpal
Capitate
Trapezoid
Hamate
Trapezium
Triquetrum
Lunate
Pisiform
Scaphoid
Ulnar styloid
Distal radioulnar joint
Radius
Ulnar

● Intermetacarpal joints
◉ Carpometacarpal joints
○ Intercarpal joints

Fig. 3.1 *The bones and joints of the wrist and hand*

Move

Examination of passive and active movement of the wrist and digits is important to determine if any weakness or fixed deformity is present. Formal assessment of grip and pinch grip srength may sometimes be of value.

Table 3.1 Normal range of movement: wrist

Extension	0–70 degrees
Flexion	0–80 degrees
Radial deviation	0–20 degrees
Ulnar deviation	0–30 degrees

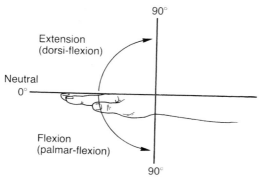

Fig. 3.2 *Flexion and extension of the wrist*

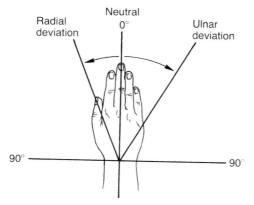

Fig. 3.3 *Radial and ulnar deviation of the wrist*

Table 3.2 Normal range of movement: fingers

Flexion	
DIP joint	0–90 degrees
PIP joint	0–100 degrees
MCP joint	0–90 degrees

Table 3.3 Normal range of movement: thumb

Flexion	
IP joint	0–80 degrees
MCP joint	0–50 degrees
CMC joint	0–15 degrees
Abduction	0–70 degrees

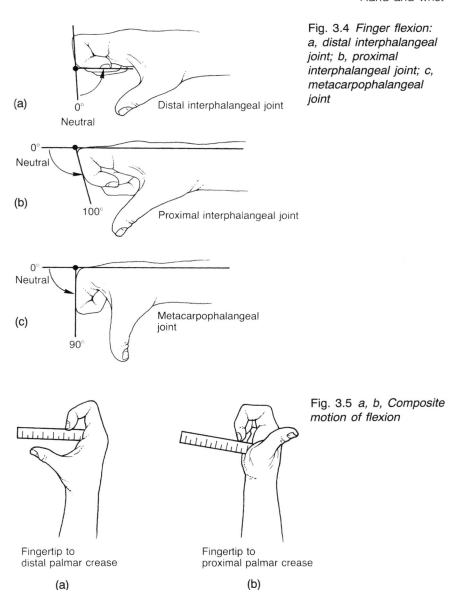

Fig. 3.4 *Finger flexion: a, distal interphalangeal joint; b, proximal interphalangeal joint; c, metacarpophalangeal joint*

(a)
0° Neutral
Distal interphalangeal joint

(b)
0° Neutral
100°
Proximal interphalangeal joint

(c)
0° Neutral
90°
Metacarpophalangeal joint

Fig. 3.5 *a, b, Composite motion of flexion*

Fingertip to distal palmar crease

(a)

Fingertip to proximal palmar crease

(b)

Common hand problems

Carpal tunnel syndrome

The diagnosis is usually clear from the history of nocturnal pain and paraesthesiae affecting a middle-aged female, though ladies of any age, and men, may be affected. There may be no physical signs, but thenar wasting, weakness or sensory impairment are indications for referral.

35

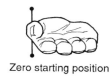

Zero starting position

Fig. 3.6 *Thumb movements:*
(a) Extension
(b) Opposition
(c) Flexion

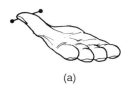

(a)

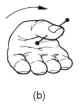

(b)

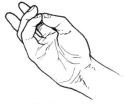

Flexion to tip of
little finger

or

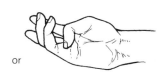

Flexion to base of
little finger

(c)

Treatment in primary care should include:

Rest — Avoid provoking activities if possible.

Night splintage — Prevents wrist flexion during sleep (flexion increases pressure in the carpal tunnel). Use a Futuro or similar splint.

Diuretics — May be helpful if fluid retention is likely.

Steroid injection — Consider injection. Eighty per cent of patients respond, but 80% recur at 2 years. Recurrence is less likely if the history is short. Most useful when resolution can be expected (pregnancy, thyroid disease). Do not inject into the median nerve.

Indications for referral are: thenar wasting or constant sensory impairment, moderate symptoms without objective neurological loss, after a 3-month trial of non-operative treatment, and severe symptoms without neurological loss.

Table 3.4 Common causes of wrist and hand pain in different age groups

Age group	Cause		
	Intra-articular	Periarticular	Referred
Childhood (2–10 years)	Infection	Fracture Osteomyelitis	
Adolescence (10–18 years)	Infection	Trauma Osteomyelitis Tumours Ganglion Idiopathic wrist pain	
Early adulthood (18–30 years)	Inflammatory arthritis Infection	Peripheral nerve entrapment Tendonitis Ganglion	Cervical
Adulthood (30–50 years)	Inflammatory arthritis Infection Osteoarthritis	Peripheral nerve entrapment Tendonitis	Cervical Chest Cardiac
Old age (>50 years)	Inflammatory arthritis Osteoarthritis	Peripheral nerve entrapment Tendonitis	Cervical Chest Cardiac

Trigger finger/thumb

Trigger finger is characterized by locking or catching of a digit during active flexion. It may be associated with rheumatoid arthritis and diabetes. Treatment in primary care should include night splintage of the interphalangeal joints in extension (a tongue depressor and tape will suffice) and steroid injection of the flexor tendon sheath. About 70% of trigger digits are asymptomatic 1 year after a single injection. Indications for referral are persistent or recurrent triggering after one injection or doubt about the diagnosis.

De Quervain's tenosynovitis

This presents with pain and swelling over the styloid process of the radius, usually after strenuous activity, and is due to inflammation of the abductor pollicis tendon sheath. Pain is aggravated by active extension of the thumb. Finkelstein's test causes pain (thumb is flexed into the palm and grasped by the fingers; the examiner moves the wrist into ulnar deviation), but should be compared to the normal side.

Treatment in primary care should include:

Rest   –   Avoid provoking activities if possible.

Splintage   –   The splint should include the thumb – a simple wrist splint is not effective.

NSAIDs   –

Steroid injection   –   Highly effective. Avoid placing steroid in the subcutaneous tissues, where it may cause atrophy.

Ganglion

1. Dorsal wrist ganglion, over the scapholunate ligament.
2. Palmar wrist ganglion, adjacent to the radial artery.
3. Palmar digital ganglion, from the flexor tendon sheath at the base of the finger.

Ganglia are common and harmless. About 40% resolve spontaneously over 10 years. Teenagers and young adults are most often affected. Patients seek advice because of pain, an unsightly swelling or concern over the diagnosis. Pain and swelling often fluctuate.

Many patients with ganglia require only explanation and reassurance that the lesion is harmless and that it may resolve spontaneously. Surgical scars at the wrist may be unattractive and excision does not always relieve pain. The recurrence rate after surgery is about 5–10% for dorsal wrist ganglia, 30% for ganglia adjacent to the radial artery and close to zero for palmar digital ganglion.

Treatment in primary care should involve explanation and reassurance. Aspiration of wrist ganglia is also possible. About 40% disappear for at least 12 months after aspiration with a wide bore needle under local anaesthesia.

For puncture of palmar digital ganglia with a 21-gauge needle, recurrence is less than 25%.

Indications for referral are large or persistently painful dorsal wrist ganglion. Indications for excision of palmar wrist ganglion are limited, as the recurrence rate approaches 30%. Painful palmar digital ganglion may persist or recur after needle puncture and require excision.

Wrist pain

There are many causes of wrist pain, some of which need surgical management. In most cases, pain is self-limiting and responds to simple measures such as support bandaging, rest, analgesics and physiotherapy. Referral is appropriate only if these measures have failed, or if the X-rays are abnormal. Patients who have normal movement, strong grip and normal plain radiographs seldom have surgically treatable pathology.

Treatment in primary care should include analgesics, NSAIDs, support bandaging and rest. Plain radiographs are useful in excluding underlying pathology. Indications for referral are persistent pain and abnormal plain radiographs

Osteoarthritis of basal thumb joint

This condition affects about 15% of the older female population. It is often asymptomatic. Management in primary care involves explanation and reassurance, NSAIDs and splintage. Steroid injection often helps: distract the joint by traction and walk the needle off the base of the metacarpal into the joint. The indication for referral is persistent pain, not responding to above measures.

Osteoarthritis of distal interphalangeal joint (Heberden's nodes)

Pain is uncommon. Females are much more commonly affected than males. It is often familial. Pain tends to subside with time, leaving the joints swollen and a little stiff, but good function is usually preserved.

Management in primary care involves advice and NSAIDs.

Indication for referral is persistent pain. Surgical fusion is the only satisfactory surgical option.

Dupuytren's disease

This disease is common and often hereditary. Alcohol, diabetes and anticonvulsant medication are risk factors. (Do not refer unless there is contracture.)

Treatment in primary care involves explanation and reassurance. Indications for referral are an inability to place the hand flat on the table and any contracture of the proximal interphalangeal joint.

Hand infections

Early soft tissue infections, before pus has formed, usually respond to antibiotics; the most common infecting organism is *Staphylococcus aureus*. Pain which prevents sleep indicates pus and is an indication for surgical drainage in hospital under adequate anaesthesia and with tourniquet control. Fluctuation appears late in the hand and is not useful in early diagnosis.

Failure to respond to antibiotics over 24–48 hours, or pain preventing sleep, are indications to refer to hospital. Beware of the 'cellulitis' which conceals a deeper abscess.

Any penetrating wound over a tendon sheath or joint should be regarded with suspicion. Flexor tendon sheath infection and septic arthritis develop over a few hours and can wreck the tendon or joint. These infections should be treated by urgent surgical drainage – antibiotics are only an adjunct to surgery. Animal bites and human tooth wounds are particularly liable to infection and frequently penetrate joints.

Common hand injuries

Fractures

Any hand injury which is followed by swelling or bruising may be a fracture. The only safe rule is to take an X-ray, as opportunities for treatment may be lost by delay. Most fractures need no treatment other than taping to an adjacent finger, but serious injuries cannot be distinguished from trivial injuries without X-ray.

Mallet finger

This is a loss of active extension of the distal interphalangeal joint due to traumatic rupture of the extensor tendon. The treatment is immediate splintage in extension, continued for 6 weeks. Apply a temporary splint and refer the patient.

Lacerations

Lacerations often conceal injuries to nerve and tendon which can be missed unless the appropriate physical signs are elicited. All structures passing near the laceration should be assumed to be divided until their integrity has been demonstrated by examination. If integrity cannot be demonstrated (small child, uncooperative adult), the wound should be explored in hospital.

Subungual haematoma

This problem is usually due to a crush injury which fractures the tuft of the terminal phalanx. Evacuation of the haematoma by piercing the nail with a hot wire relieves pain.

Case Histories

1

A 45-year-old woman with a 3-month history of nocturnal pain, numbness and tingling in both hands, without neurological signs.

Treatment with simple analgesics	1
NSAIDs	1
Rest	1
Referral for physiotherapy	0
Use of splints/support/bandage	1
Joint aspiration	0
Steroid injection	1
Blood test	1
X-ray	0
Routine referral	0
Urgent referral	0
Emergency referral	0
None of these	0

Response: The history suggests carpal tunnel compression. With a short history and absence of neurological signs, night splinting is appropriate.

2

A 60-year-old woman with a 2-year history of nocturnal pain, paraesthesiae and numbness in both hands. Constant numbness in thumb, index and middle fingers with thenar wasting.

Treatment with simple analgesics	1
NSAIDs	1
Rest	0
Referral for physiotherapy	0
Use of splints/support/bandage	0
Joint aspiration	0
Steroid injection	0
Blood test	1
X-ray	0
Routine referral	0
Urgent referral	1
Emergency referral	0
None of these	0

Response: Neurological signs indicate severe or prolonged carpal tunnel compression. Referral for consideration of surgery.

3

A 20-year-old female with a 12-month history of small, non-tender dorsal wrist swelling.

Treatment with simple analgesics	1
NSAIDs	0
Rest	1
Referral for physiotherapy	0
Use of splints/support/bandage	1
Joint aspiration	1
Steroid injection	0
Blood test	0
X-ray	0
Routine referral	0
Urgent referral	0
Emergency referral	0
None of these	0

Response: Dorsal wrist ganglion is harmless and may resolve without treatment. Referral appropriate if large or persistently painful.

4

A 70-year-old female with a 2-year history of pain, swelling and stiffness at the base of the right thumb.

Treatment with simple analgesics	1
NSAIDs	1
Rest	1
Referral for physiotherapy	0
Use of splints/support/bandage	1
Joint aspiration	0
Steroid injection	1
Blood test	0
X-ray	1
Routine referral	0
Urgent referral	0
Emergency referral	0
None of these	0

Response: X-ray to look for basal joint arthritis. NSAIDs or analgesics, splintage and injection. Referral for persistent symptoms.

5

A 45-year-old male with a 6-week history of painful locking of the ring finger in flexion.

Treatment with simple analgesics	1
NSAIDs	1
Rest	1
Referral for physiotherapy	0
Use of splints/support/bandage	0
Joint aspiration	0
Steroid injection	1
Blood test	0
X-ray	0
Routine referral	1
Urgent referral	0
Emergency referral	0
None of these	0

Response: Seventy per cent of trigger fingers respond to steroid injection. Routine referral if locking persists.

6

A 55-year-old male with a 12-month history of pain and stiffness at the right wrist. Movement reduced by 50%.

Treatment with simple analgesics	1
NSAIDs	1
Rest	1
Referral for physiotherapy	0
Use of splints/support/bandage	1
Joint aspiration	0
Steroid injection	0
Blood test	0
X-ray	1
Routine referral	1
Urgent referral	0
Emergency referral	0
None of these	0

Response: X-ray to exclude osteoarthritis. NSAIDs and splintage. Routine referral if pain persists.

7

A 35-year-old male with a 48-hour history of acute pain (preventing sleep), swelling and stiffness of the thumb metacarpal joint after pruning roses.

Treatment with simple analgesics	0
NSAIDs	0
Rest	0
Referral for physiotherapy	0
Use of splints/support/bandage	0
Joint aspiration	1
Steroid injection	0
Blood test	1
X-ray	1
Routine referral	0
Urgent referral	0
Emergency referral	1
None of these	0

Response: Emergency referral to exclude septic arthritis.

8

A 70-year-old male with a 12-month history of linear subcutaneous thickening in the right palm.

Treatment with simple analgesics	0
NSAIDs	0
Rest	0
Referral for physiotherapy	0
Use of splints/support/bandage	0
Joint aspiration	0
Steroid injection	0
Blood test	0
X-ray	0
Routine referral	0
Urgent referral	0
Emergency referral	0
None of these	1

Response: Dupuytren's disease. Referral only if contracture develops.

9

A 40-year-old male with a 4-week history of pain, swelling and tenderness over abductor pollicis longus tendon sheath in the right wrist.

Treatment with simple analgesics	1
NSAIDs	1
Rest	1
Referral for physiotherapy	1
Use of splints/support/bandage	1
Joint aspiration	0
Steroid injection	1
Blood test	0
X-ray	0
Routine referral	0
Urgent referral	0
Emergency referral	0
None of these	0

Response: De Quervain's tenosynovitis. Splint, NSAIDs, with or without steroid injection. Refer if injection fails.

10

A 60-year-old female with rheumatoid arthritis notices sudden loss of active extension of her right ring and little fingers.

Treatment with simple analgesics	0
NSAIDs	0
Rest	0
Referral for physiotherapy	0
Use of splints/support/bandage	1
Joint aspiration	0
Steroid injection	0
Blood test	0
X-ray	1
Routine referral	0
Urgent referral	1
Emergency referral	0
None of these	0

Response: Extensor tendon rupture. Other ruptures may follow without warning. Urgent referral.

Injection of the base of the thumb

Indications

For arthritis of the carpometacarpal joint.

Technique

Palpate the extensor pollicis and abductor pollicis longus tendons at the base of the thumb metacarpal. Then palpate the joint at the base of the metacarpal just anterior to these tendons. Insert a 2-gauge needle onto the metacarpal and 'walk' the needle into the joint. Insert to a depth of 5–8 mm and inject gradually.

Usually use 2 ml of a combination of **either** 10–25 mg hydrocortisone acetate, **or** 500 mg triamcinalone, **or** 10–20 mg methylprednisolone with 1% lidocaine.

Frequency

Every 4–6 weeks. If there is no benefit after two to three injections then consider alternative treatment or referral.

Structures at risk

Injection directly onto bone or periosteum is exquisitely painful, so try and avoid it.

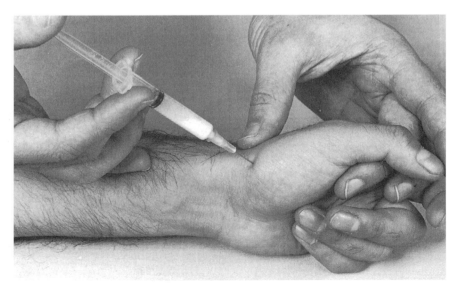

Fig. 3.7 *Injection into the base of the thumb*

Injection for De Quervain's tenosynovitis

Indications

For stenosing tenosynovitis of the abductor pollicis longus and extensor pollicis brevis tendons over the radial styloid (De Quervain's).

Technique

Palpate the dorsal aspect of the radial styloid, there is normally a thickened tendon sheath. As the thumb moves crepitus may be felt. Insert a 21-gauge needle in the line of the tendons into the tendon sheath to a depth of 3–5 mm and inject gradually.

Usually use 1 ml of 10–25 mg hydrocortisone acetate.

Frequency

Every 4–6 weeks. If there is no benefit after two to three injections then consider alternative treatment or referral.

Structures at risk

Also avoid injecting under pressure into tendon as there is a theoretical risk of causing tendon damage. Depot and subcutaneous injections may cause unsightly fat atrophy.

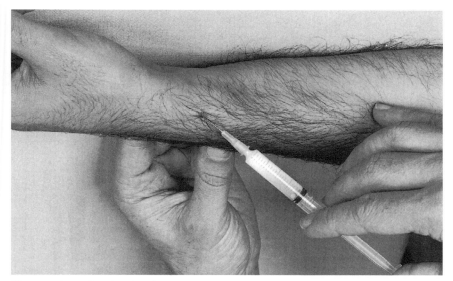

Fig. 3.8 *Insertion for De Quervain's tenosynovitis*

Injection of the carpal tunnel

Indications

Carpal tunnel syndrome.

Technique

Identify the distal wrist creases and insert a 19-gauge needle. 1 cm proximal to the crease, mid-way between the tendons of palmarus longus and flexor carpi ulnaris. Inject 1 ml of saline or L.A. if no pain or paraesthesiae are felt, then inject 1 ml of a combination of **either** 10–25 mg hydrocortisone acetate, **or** 5–10 mg triamcinalone, **or** 10–20 mg methylprednisolone with 1% lidocaine.

Frequency

If there is no benefit after one injection then refer.

Structures at risk

The median nerve is obviously at risk. If there are any symptoms of pain or paraesthesiae radiating into the fingers or thumb then you should stop injecting. Steroid injection into the median nerve may cause permanent damage.

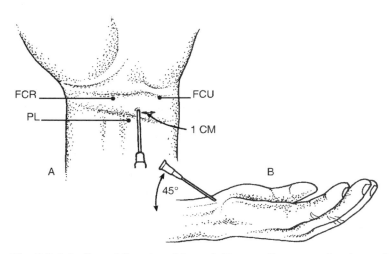

Fig. 3.9 *Injection of the carpal tunnel. The median nerve lies beneath the tendon of palmaris longus (PL). The ulnar nerve lies beneath the tendon of flexor carpi ulnaris (FCU). The safe corridor for injection is midway between these tendons*

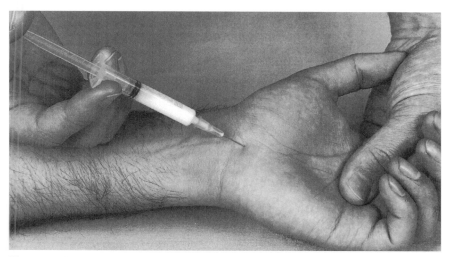

Fig. 3.10 *Injection of the carpal tunnel*

Injection into the palm for trigger finger or thumb

Indications

For trigger finger or thumb.

Technique

Palpate the nodule of the flexor tendon. This lies about 1 cm proximal to the level of the web space.

Using a 21-gauge needle inject from proximal to distal to a depth of 3–6 mm. Inject around the nodule into the tendon sheath. Do not inject against resistance into the tendon.

Usually use 1–2 ml of a combination of **either** 10–25 mg hydrocortisone acetate, **or** 5–10 mg triamcinalone, **or** 10–20 mg methylprednisolone with 1% lidocaine.

Frequency

Every 4–6 weeks. If there is no benefit after two injections then consider referral.

Structures at risk

Avoid injecting under pressure into tendon as there is a theoretical risk of causing tendon damage.

The digital nerves lie on either side of the tendon. Injection over the nodule and in the line of the tendon should be safe.

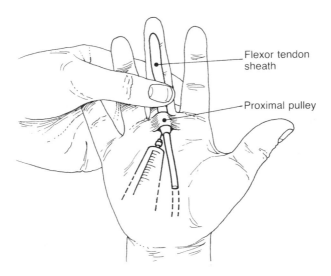

Fig. 3.11 *Injection into the palm for trigger finger or thumb*

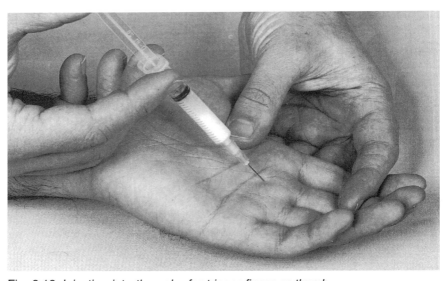

Fig. 3.12 *Injection into the palm for trigger finger or thumb*

Further reading

Green, D. P. (1984). Diagnostic and therapeutic value of carpal tunnel injection. *J Hand Surg*, **9A**; 850–854.

McGrath, M. M. (1984). Local steroid therapy in the hand. *J Hand Surg*, **9A**; 915–921.

4

Cervical spineJeremy C. T. Fairbank

- Neck instability is an important symptom usually reflecting serious pathology.
- Most patients with cervical spondylosis respond to conservative treatment.
- A patient with a history of trauma and neck symptoms who has already had a cervical spine X-ray, may require a further X-ray examination.
- Sixty per cent of whiplash injuries respond within 3 months – litigation has an adverse effect on outcome.

Presenting symptoms

Neck problems may present with pain, stiffness, neurological deficit, and occasionally clicking, snapping or sensations of 'instability'.

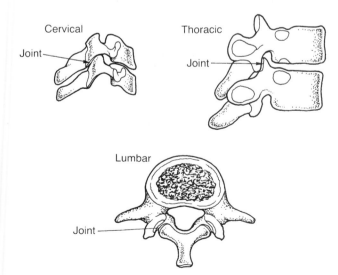

Fig. 4.1 *Regional differences between vertebrae*

Pain

Pain is commonly intermittent and related to activity.

Rest pain or night pain should be taken seriously and may be due to tumour or infection. It is an indication for taking a plain radiograph.

Pain may be experienced in the midline, and may also be referred distally (usually no more than two segments). Pain may be referred out into the shoulders and arms by two mechanisms. One is the familiar **root pain** where symptoms are experienced in typical dermatomal distribution. The other is **referred pain**, which is much less easy to define, although extremely commonly experienced. This is frequently felt in the shoulder or upper arm and tends to radiate further down the arm the worse the pain is. This pain is referred in a 'sclerodermal' fashion in the distribution of the innervation of muscle. This phenomenon occurs in pain arising in all parts of the spine but is particularly obvious in pain arising from the neck and low back. Referred pain may be accompanied by local tenderness at the source of radiating pain as well as in the distribution of that pain. These 'trigger points' have also been called 'fibrosis' or 'tender points' and can be helped on occasion by injections of local anaesthetic or dry needling (acupuncture).

Pain may develop acutely or chronically. Patients always have difficulty in describing pain, but it may be experienced in the distributions described above. It is worth examining the cervical spine for tenderness to see whether or not you can reproduce pain from a specific level. You may also find tender points distributed over the back scapulae, shoulders or in the arms. How important these tender points are remains controversial and is certainly not an essential part of the examination. Pain from the neck is sometimes difficult to distinguish clinically from pain arising from the shoulder or arm. Usually movement of the shoulder, elbow or wrist may reproduce the pain and draw one's attention away from the cervical spine as a source of that pain.

Stiffness

This frequently, but not always, accompanies pain. This is not usually of diagnostic significance, but may relate to the patient's perception of disability.

Neurological symptoms and signs

Pain, paraesthesia, weakness and loss of function may present in a dermatomal distribution. This often, although not always, reflects significant neurological damage, and must always be taken seriously. Cervical myelopathy may present insidiously and is not always easy to diagnose.

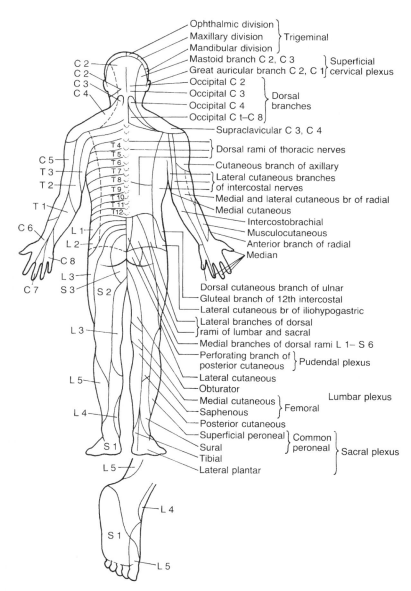

Fig. 4.2 *Dermatomes (cutaneous distribution of spinal segments and peripheral nerves): posterior aspect*

There may be difficulties with walking and unsteadiness on the feet. In the upper limbs, pain, weakness and loss of dexterity may be experienced. The classic dermatomes are illustrated in Figure 4.2. The distribution of motor signs relating to nerve roots is shown in Figure 4.3.

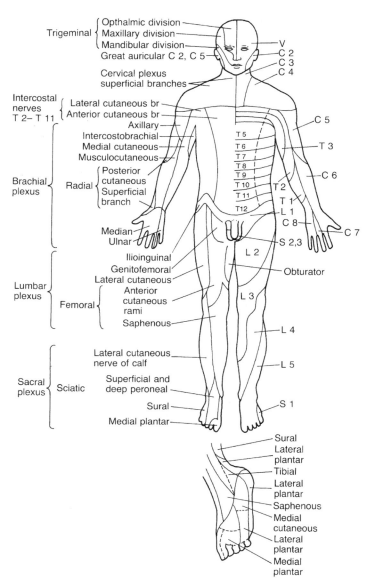

Fig. 4.3 *Dermatomes (cutaneous distribution of spinal segments and peripheral nerves): anterior aspect*

Patients with cervical myelopathy may exhibit Lehmitte's sign which is a sensation of 'electric shocks' on flexion or extension of the neck. These electric shocks or paraesthesia may be experienced in all four limbs as well as over the top of the head. There may be disturbance of the normal deep tendon relaxes and occasionally you may find a positive Hoffman's sign (flicking of the volar surface of the middle finger causes flexion of the thumb and index finger). Bladder and bowl dysfunction should be enquired after, but is not always experienced in patients with chronic myelopathy.

Instability

This occurs when the neck is rendered unstable by trauma, tumours or destructive arthropathies (rheumatoid osteoarthritis, fractures in ankylosing spondylitis, etc.). This symptom must always be taken seriously.

Instability means a sensation that the patient does not normally experience. Patients feels that their head is no longer firmly fixed to the rest of the body, or that any movements engender a sensation of panic. At its extreme, patients may support their head with their hands. Patients may have difficulties in describing symptoms, particularly if they are something new and unfamiliar. On occasion neck pain may be associated with sensations of dizziness.

Physical examination

Look for position and range of movement of the cervical spine, as well as torticollis and muscle wasting.

Neurological examination

Perform a neurological examination of the upper limbs, and always include tests of sensation, power and reflexes. If you suspect cervical spine pathology then also observe the gait and examine the neurology of the legs.

A rapid screen of the upper limbs involves resisted abduction of the shoulder, flexion and extension of the elbow, dorsiflexion of the wrist, abduction of the fingers and abduction of the thumbs.

Table 4.1 Normal range of movement: neck

Flexion	0–45 degrees
Extension	0–45 degrees
Lateral flexion	0–45 degrees
Rotation	0–60 degrees

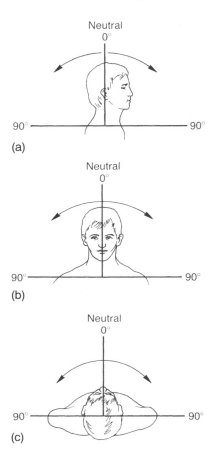

Neutral
0°

90° ———— 90°

(a)

Neutral
0°

90° ———— 90°

(b)

Neutral
0°

90° ———— 90°

(c)

Fig. 4.4 *a, Flexion; b, lateral flexion; c, rotation*

General management principles

If there is a clear-cut history of trauma, then obtain an X-ray to exclude bony pathology and refer for physiotherapy assessment. You should not be afraid of requesting a further X-ray if a patient has already had a radiograph in any department, as late subluxation from soft tissue injuries to the neck is well recognized and sometimes fractures are missed at the initial examination. In case of doubt refer to an orthopaedic surgeon.

If there is no history of trauma and the pain is intermittent, consider NSAIDs and treat with a soft collar and physiotherapy if there is no response to anti-inflammatories. A soft collar is sometimes best worn at night and it is worth the patient experimenting with this. As far as possible one should avoid prolonged immobilization in the collar.

If the pain is continuous with night pain, request a radiograph and consider tumour and infection. This may be an indication for referral to a specialist.

If there are definite signs or definite neurological symptoms, obtain an X-ray (and MRI if you have access) and refer to an orthopaedic surgeon.

Sensations of instability should be taken seriously and it is probably an indication for urgent referral to an orthopaedic surgeon.

Common cervical problems

Torticollis

This may been seen in infants, and normally responds to stretching by the mother under physiotherapy supervision. In older children and adults it may occur spontaneously or after a minor injury (acute rotatory subluxation). There is a spectrum of complaints, from the trivial which can be managed by reassurance and rest, to more severe symptoms which should probably be referred to a specialist. A very severe torticollis responds to inpatient traction and physiotherapy and is, therefore, an indication for emergency referral. Some patients with minor stiffness will respond to manipulative treatment from the physiotherapist or a qualified alternative practitioner.

Cervical spondylosis

This is a generic term which covers a wide range of common disorders of the cervical spine secondary to degenerative changes in the cervical intervertebral discs and their adjacent synovial joints (the joints of Luschka). These joints are exclusively present in the neck and are one of the reasons why rheumatoid arthritis produces serious problems in the cervical spine, but not so commonly elsewhere in the spine. The facet or apophyseal joints are synovial and are also involved in rheumatoid arthritis. Cervical spondylosis is frequently asymptomatic and may be detected by minor changes on plain radiographs. In some patients the chronicity and severity of pain may be an indication for referral if simple measures such as a collar, non-steroidals or physiotherapy are ineffective. In more severe cases this process may cause nerve root pain by nerve root irritation and compression. In the worst circumstances, particularly if the patient has the misfortune to be born with a narrow cervical canal, then it may cause cervical myelopathy, as described above. Most patients with cervical spondylosis would respond to conservative measures and do not require specialist referral. There are a small minority of patients with chronic cervical pain who respond to cervical fusion, usually performed from the front of the neck. This operation also allows nerve root decompression, although this can be performed from behind. Depending on local circumstances, this may be performed by neurosurgeons or orthopaedic surgeons. Cervical spondylosis may be a cause of

Table 4.2 Primary management of cervical spondylosis associated with arm pain

Advice and education	Reassurance
	Rest
	Occupation
	Psychotherapy
Physiotherapy	Heat/cold
Chiropractic	Exercises
Osteopathy	Acupuncture
	TENS
	Traction
Drugs	Analgesics
	NSAIDs
	Injections

headaches but this symptom should be handled within the normal differential diagnosis for headaches and is outside the scope of this book. On occasion a radiograph may be of therapeutic value to explain the process to patients and to reassure them.

Cervical fractures

Whilst the majority of these are recognized acutely and are managed by the emergency services, diagnosis of serious injury may be delayed because:

1 the original injury was missed;
2 the severity only becomes apparent after the general practitioner has requested a radiograph, usually because of persisting or increasing pain;
3 a late deformity has developed;
4 there is a progressive neurological deficit. These patients require immediate referral for specialist management, usually by an orthopaedic surgeon.

Whiplash or soft tissue injury to the neck

Neck pain is common to victims of road traffic accidents, particularly after rear-end collisions. Whilst this may start acutely, it often starts within hours or a day after the injury. This is a common reason for consultation in primary care. In some patients low back pain may start at a later stage. The pathology of these injuries is not understood in spite of considerable research. At least 60% of cases will resolve within 3

Table 4.3 Factors associated with persistent and severe whiplash injuries

Severe whiplash injury

High-speed injury
Intense and rapid onset of pain
Severe restriction of movement at presentation
Abnormal neurology
Bony injuries

Persistent whiplash injury

High-speed injury
Intense and rapid onset of pain
Severe restriction of movement at presentation
Abnormal neurology
Bony injuries
Increasing age
Upper limb paraesthesiae
Cervical spondylosis

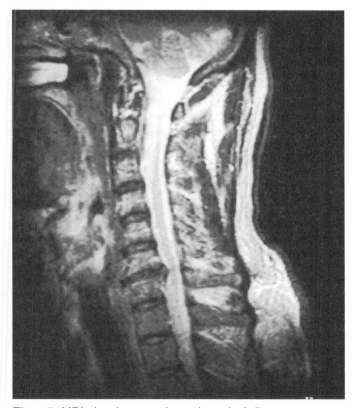

Fig. 4.5 *MRI showing a prolapsed cervical disc*

months. In the rest, symptoms will tend to improve until they stabilize 1 year from the injuries. The management of these injuries is controversial but some benefit may be obtained from physiotherapy and a soft collar at night. Plain radiograph is indicated in the early stage to detect a fracture but this investigation is invariably normal. Severe persisting pain may be an indication for specialist referral after 6 months if the neck has been cleared by simple radiograph postinjury. These cases almost invariably involve litigation and litigation has an adverse effect on the outcome.

Cervical disc prolapse

This is less common than a lumbar disc prolapse. It usually affects the central segments of the cervical spine. Root pain is usually preceded by a variable period of neck pain. Neurological signs in the distribution of the affected nerve root may be present. In most cases these settle down with analgesics and the symptoms resolve. There is a controversial place for steroids if the pain persists. If there is a progressive neurological deficit, seek a specialist opinion.

Case Histories

1

A 4-year-old child falls out of bed. The next morning his mother notices that he has a painless torticollis.

Simple analgesics	1
NSAIDs	0
Rest	0
Physiotherapy	0
Splints/support/bandages	0
Aspiration	0
Steroid injection	0
Blood test	0
X-ray	0
Routine referral	0
Urgent referral	1
Emergency referral	0
None of these	0

Answer: Probably acute rotatory subluxation. If it is painful or persists, this requires specialist management

2

A 35-year-old female develops chronic neck pain without referral or neurological signs. The pain is of variable intensity.

Simple analgesics	1
NSAIDs	1
Rest	0
Physiotherapy	1
Splints/support/bandages	0
Aspiration	0
Steroid injection	0
Blood test	0
X-ray	0
Routine referral	0
Urgent referral	0
Emergency referral	0
None of these	0

Answer: Non-specific neck pain, often, but not always associated with cervical spondylosis. This may resolve rapidly with symptomatic treatment. If it does not resolve rapidly, refer for physiotherapy.

3

A 35-year-old female develops continuous pain without referral which wakes her at night and is of unremitting intensity.

Simple analgesics	1
NSAIDs	1
Rest	0
Physiotherapy	1
Splints/support/bandages	0
Aspiration	0
Steroid injection	0
Blood test	1
X-ray	1
Routine referral	1
Urgent referral	1
Emergency referral	0
None of these	0

Answer: Unremitting pain may be a manifestation of 'illness behaviour', but should always be taken seriously. If pain persists, a plain X-ray may be helpful in eliminating serious pathology. Seek specialist help if it does not resolve. How long to wait before seeking advice depends on clinical assessment.

4

A woman of 47 develops neck pain followed by arm pain and paraesthesiae. Later she develops weakness of wrist dorsiflexion.

Simple analgesics	1
NSAIDs	1
Rest	0
Physiotherapy	0
Splints/support/bandages	0
Aspiration	0
Steroid injection	0
Blood test	0
X-ray	1
Routine referral	0
Urgent referral	1
Emergency referral	1
None of these	0

Answer: Cervical root irritation due to disc or spondylosis is the most likely. These symptoms can resolve spontaneously, but surgery may be indicated if investigation confirms the diagnosis. Plain X-rays are not much help here, but can sometimes show pathology.

Further reading

An, H, and Simpson, J. M. (1994). *Surgery of the Cervical Spine.* Martin Dunitz, London.

Grieve, G. (1994). *Musculoskeletal Mobilisation: The Spine.* Churchill Livingstone, Edinburgh.

Jeffrey, E. (ed.) (1993). *Disorders of the Cervical Spine,* 2nd edn. Butterworth-Heinemann, Oxford.

5

Lumbar spine ___ James Wilson-MacDonald

- Mechanical low back pain is best treated by early mobilization and physiotherapy.
- Back pain which is unremitting or associated with urinary and bowel symptoms, or weakness requires urgent referral.
- Twenty per cent of asymptomatic individuals will have evidence of disc prolapse on an MRI scan.
- Characteristic features of spinal stenosis in the elderly include leg pain induced by walking, relieved by sitting and associated with numbness and paraesthesiae.

Presenting symptoms

It is important to differentiate between the conditions which require acute referral and conditions where conservative measures such as physiotherapy should be used prior to referral.

Pain and neurological symptoms

Symptoms which may require urgent referral include night pain of a constant nature, constant unremitting pain, urinary or bowel symptoms, or symptoms of weakness. Constant unremitting pain is suggestive either of malignancy or of infection, and these patients are best seen as early as possible. Referral either immediately or within a few days is indicated, depending on the severity of the symptoms. Patients who present with weakness in the limbs or with urological or bowel symptoms may have compression either of the nerve root or of the spinal cord, urgent referral is indicated.

Chronic pain

The more chronic symptoms which most patients present with, such as low back pain, mild neurological symptoms in the legs or intermittent neurological symptoms in the legs, do not require such urgent referral, indeed most of these patients benefit from a period of delay in that many

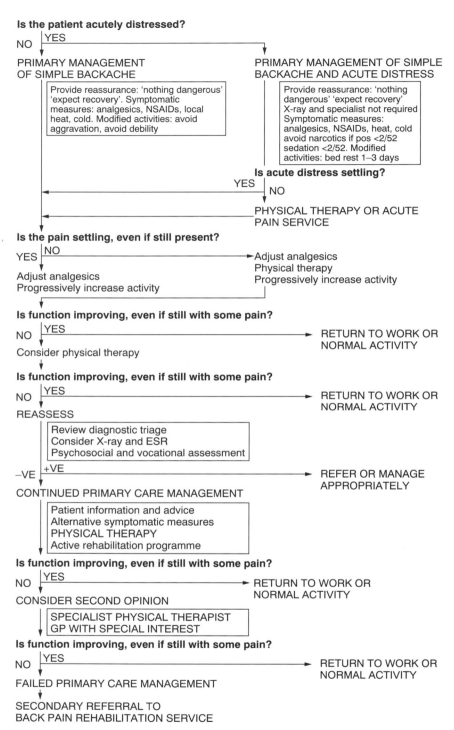

Is the patient acutely distressed?

NO | YES

PRIMARY MANAGEMENT
OF SIMPLE BACKACHE

> Provide reassurance: 'nothing dangerous'
> 'expect recovery'. Symptomatic
> measures: analgesics, NSAIDs, local
> heat, cold. Modified activities: avoid
> aggravation, avoid debility

PRIMARY MANAGEMENT OF SIMPLE
BACKACHE AND ACUTE DISTRESS

> Provide reassurance: 'nothing
> dangerous' 'expect recovery'
> X-ray and specialist not required
> Symptomatic measures:
> analgesics, NSAIDs, heat, cold
> avoid narcotics if pos <2/52
> sedation <2/52. Modified
> activities: bed rest 1–3 days

Is acute distress settling?

YES | NO

PHYSICAL THERAPY OR ACUTE
PAIN SERVICE

Is the pain settling, even if still present?

YES | NO

Adjust analgesics
Progressively increase activity

Adjust analgesics
Physical therapy
Progressively increase activity

Is function improving, even if still with some pain?

NO | YES → RETURN TO WORK OR NORMAL ACTIVITY

Consider physical therapy

Is function improving, even if still with some pain?

NO | YES → RETURN TO WORK OR NORMAL ACTIVITY

REASSESS

> Review diagnostic triage
> Consider X-ray and ESR
> Psychosocial and vocational assessment

–VE | +VE → REFER OR MANAGE APPROPRIATELY

CONTINUED PRIMARY CARE MANAGEMENT

> Patient information and advice
> Alternative symptomatic measures
> PHYSICAL THERAPY
> Active rehabilitation programme

Is function improving, even if still with some pain?

NO | YES → RETURN TO WORK OR NORMAL ACTIVITY

CONSIDER SECOND OPINION

> SPECIALIST PHYSICAL THERAPIST
> GP WITH SPECIAL INTEREST

Is function improving, even if still with some pain?

NO | YES → RETURN TO WORK OR NORMAL ACTIVITY

FAILED PRIMARY CARE MANAGEMENT

SECONDARY REFERRAL TO
BACK PAIN REHABILITATION SERVICE

Fig. 5.1 *Primary care management of simple backache. (Adapted from Clinical Standards Advisory Group, 1994)*

Initial consultation

Diagnostic triage
- simple backache
- nerve root pain ⎱ urgent
- serious spinal pathology ⎰ referral

Early management strategy:

Aims: symptomatic relief of pain; prevent disability

Prescribe simple analgesia, NSAIDs
- avoid narcotics if possible and never more than two weeks

Arrange physical therapy if symptoms last more than a few days
- manipulation
- active exercise and physical activity
  - modifies pain mechanisms, speeds recovery

Advise rest only if essential: 1–3 days
- prolonged bed rest is harmful

Encourage early activity
- activity is not harmful
- reduces pain
- physical fitness beneficial

Practise psychosocial management; this is fundamental
- promote positive attitudes to activity and work
- distress and depression

Advise absence from work only if unavoidable; early return to work
- prolonged sickness absence makes return to work increasingly difficult

Biopsychosocial assessment at 6 weeks

Review diagnostic triage
ESR and X-ray lumbosacral spine if specifically indicated
Psychosocial and vocational assessment

Active rehabilitation programme

Incremental aerobic exercise and fitness programme of physical reconditioning
Behavioural medicine principles
Close liaison with the workplace

Secondary referral

Second opinion
Rehabilitation
Vocational assessment and guidance
Surgery
Pain management

Final outcome measure: maintain productive activity; reduce work loss

Fig. 5.2 *Overview of management guidelines for acute back pain. (Adapted from Clinical Standards Advisory Group, 1994)*

of them resolve spontaneously. Conservative treatment especially in the form of physiotherapy may make referral unnecessary. Every patient referred to hospital with mechanical low back pain should have had physiotherapy prior to referral to hospital.

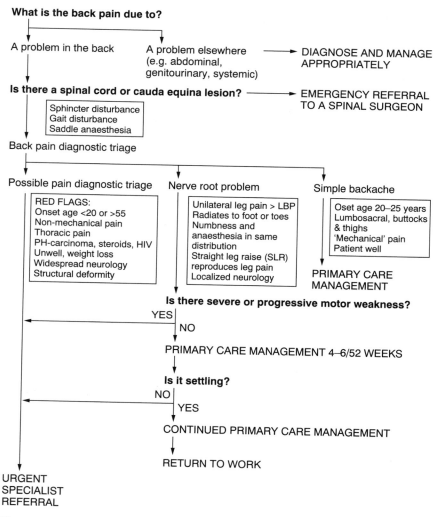

What is the back pain due to?

A problem in the back

A problem elsewhere (e.g. abdominal, genitourinary, systemic) ⟶ DIAGNOSE AND MANAGE APPROPRIATELY

Is there a spinal cord or cauda equina lesion? ⟶ EMERGENCY REFERRAL TO A SPINAL SURGEON

Sphincter disturbance
Gait disturbance
Saddle anaesthesia

Back pain diagnostic triage

Possible pain diagnostic triage

Nerve root problem

Simple backache

RED FLAGS:
Onset age <20 or >55
Non-mechanical pain
Thoracic pain
PH-carcinoma, steroids, HIV
Unwell, weight loss
Widespread neurology
Structural deformity

Unilateral leg pain > LBP
Radiates to foot or toes
Numbness and
anaesthesia in same
distribution
Straight leg raise (SLR)
reproduces leg pain
Localized neurology

Oset age 20–25 years
Lumbosacral, buttocks
& thighs
'Mechanical' pain
Patient well

PRIMARY CARE MANAGEMENT

Is there severe or progressive motor weakness?

YES | NO

PRIMARY CARE MANAGEMENT 4–6/52 WEEKS

Is it settling?

NO | YES

CONTINUED PRIMARY CARE MANAGEMENT

RETURN TO WORK

URGENT SPECIALIST REFERRAL

Fig. 5.3 *Diagnostic triage of a patient presenting with low back pain with or without sciatica. (Adapted from Clinical Standards Advisory Group, 1994)*

Physical examination

Look

Observation of the way the patient moves about and dresses and undresses is helpful in confirming the severity of symptoms. Observation of the back may reveal muscle spasm or a deformity of the spine. Often the deformity is due to a so-called sciatic scoliosis; when

SIMPLE BACKACHE

Onset generally age 20–55 years
Lumbosacral region, buttocks and thighs
Pain 'mechanical' in nature
 – varies with physical activity
 – varies with time
Patient well
Prognosis good
 –90% recover from acute attack in 6 weeks

RED FLAGS

Possible serious spinal pathology

Age of onset <25 or >55 years
Violent trauma: e.g. fall from a height, RTA
Constant, progressive, non-mechanical pain
Thoracic pain
Post medical history – carcinoma
Systemic steroids
Drug abuse, HIV
Systemically unwell
Weight loss
Persisting severe restriction of lumbar flexion
Widespread neurology
Structural deformity

If there are suspicious clinical features or if pain has not settled in 6 weeks, an ESR and plain X-ray should be considered.

NERVE ROOT PAIN

Unilateral leg pain > back pain
Pain generally radiates to foot to toes
Numbness and paraesthesia in the same distribution
Nerve irritation signs
 – reduced straight leg raise which reproduces leg pain
Motor, sensory or reflex change
 – limited to one nerve root
Prognosis reasonable
 – 50% recover from acute attack within 6 weeks

CAUDA EQUINA SYNDROME/WIDESPREAD NEUROLOGICAL DISORDER

Difficulty with micturition
Loss of anal spincter tone or faecal incontinence
Saddle anaesthesia about the anus, perineum or genitals
Widespread (>one nerve root) or progressive motor weakness in the legs or gait disturbance

INFLAMMATORY DISORDERS

Ankylosing spondylitis and related disorders

Gradual onset
Marked morning stiffness
Persisting limitation of spinal movements in all directions
Peripheral joint involvement
Iritis, skin rashes (psoriasis), colitis, urethral discharge
Family history

Fig. 5.4 *Diagnostic indicators for simple backache, nerve root pain, red flags, cauda equina syndrome and inflammatory disorders. (Adapted from Clinical Standards Advisory Group, 1994)*

the patient lies down, the deformity resolves. Fixed deformities are suggestive of scoliosis or severe degenerative changes. There may be muscle wasting in the lower limbs, although this is unusual except in chronic conditions.

Palpate

Palpation will reveal the area of tenderness in the spine, and it helps to some extent with isolating the level of the lesion.

Move

Sciatic and femoral stretch test may be positive if there is nerve root compression. The femoral stretch test is performed with the patient prone, knee flexed and when the hip is extended, a positive test is elicited with pain down the front of the thigh.

Neurology

Reflex changes are also useful in isolating the level of nerve root compression, although there is considerable variation in the nerve root supply of any single reflex, and these are not necessarily reliable. Lesions such as disc prolapse may also affect more than one nerve root.

Signs of neurological impairment

If the patient has bowel or urinary symptoms, or there is significant nerve root pain or spinal cord compression is suspected, then rectal examination and examination of perineal sensation is essential. Reduced

Table 5.1 Normal range of movement: thoracolumbar spine

Flexion	0–80 degrees
Extension	0–20 degrees
Lateral bend	0–35 degrees
Rotation	0–45 degrees

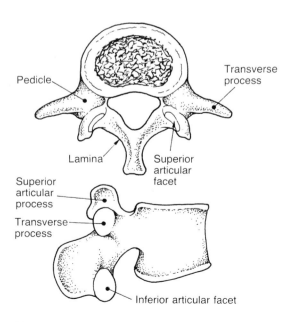

Fig. 5.5 *Anatomical features of lumbar vertebra*

anal tone or altered sensation in the perineum may be suggestive of a lesion such as a central cord lesion in the lower lumbar spine. Upper motor neurone signs in the lower limbs suggest a lesion compressing the spinal cord itself. These include upgoing plantars, clonus, difficulty with balance and weakness in the lower limbs.

Inappropriate signs

Waddell has described various inappropriate signs, and if patients exhibit these signs, it is suggested there may be some overlay and exaggeration of their symptoms. These include widespread tenderness in the spine, non-anatomical weakness, jerky movements, non-anatomical sensory disturbance, pain in the lumbar spine or in the legs felt on axial compression along the spine, and reduced straight-leg raising but the ability to sit on the bench with the knee extended and the hip fully flexed. However, these are only pointers to exaggerated behaviour and are not necessarily reliable in confirming exaggeration of symptoms.

Common spinal problems

Mechanical low back pain

Between 60 and 90% of the population will experience mechanical low back pain at some point in their lives. It often follows an episode of heavy lifting or an injury to the back. Fortunately, more than 90% of these patients have resolution of their back pain within 6 weeks of the onset. Typically they are virtually painfree at rest, but movement in bed may make the pain worse. Activities tend to aggravate the problem. Up to 3 days of bed rest may be useful, but thereafter physiotherapy is the mainstay of treatment in the early stages. Patients with mechanical back pain should only be referred to hospital if their symptoms continue for more than 6 weeks, and if the symptoms are severe enough to interfere significantly with day-to-day activities or if the patient is unable to work. Invasive treatments are not usually indicated unless the patient has had significant pain for up to a year.

It is important to differentiate mechanical back pain from back pain due to infection or malignancy.

Disc prolapse

Disc prolapse is common in individuals between the age of 20 and 60. Occasionally this follows an acute incident, but usually the onset is gradual, although there may be precipitating factors. Usually the patients present initially with back pain, and then often this is followed by nerve root pain radiating down the leg usually into the calf and the

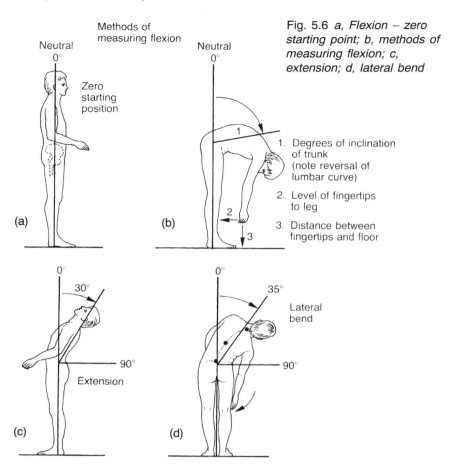

Methods of measuring flexion

Fig. 5.6 *a, Flexion – zero starting point; b, methods of measuring flexion; c, extension; d, lateral bend*

1. Degrees of inclination of trunk (note reversal of lumbar curve)
2. Level of fingertips to leg
3. Distance between fingertips and floor

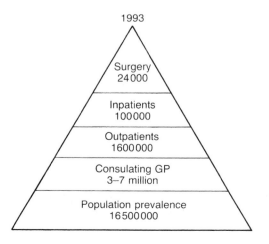

Fig. 5.7 *Estimated annual health care for back pain in 1993 (number of cases)*

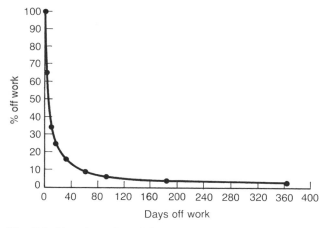

Fig. 5.8 *Duration of work loss with back pain; over 90% of sufferers will return to work within 50 days*

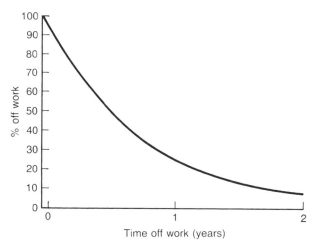

Fig. 5.9 *Probability of returning to work with increasing time off work*

foot. Fortunately 90% of individuals with a disc prolapse will have resolution of their symptoms in the first 6 weeks. Three days of bed rest may be helpful initially and early physiotherapy may also be helpful.

Indications for hospital referral are:

1 Severe uncontrollable pain.
2 Symptoms which persist more than 6 weeks and are not improving.
3 Cauda equina symptoms of urinary and bowel symptoms.
4 Weakness in the limbs.

Table 5.2 Summary of diagnostic triage and referral

	Initial management	*If not resolving by 4–6 weeks*
Possible serious spinal pathology	Urgent/emergency referral for specialist investigation	
Nerve root problem	General practitioner ? Refer for acute pain control ? Physiotherapy ?? Osteopathy/chiropractic	Urgent surgical referral
Simple backache	General practitioner ? Physiotherapy ? Osteopathy/chiropractic ?? Refer for acute pain control	Psychological and vocational assessment Active rehabilitation for return to work

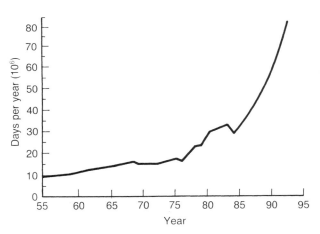

Fig. 5.10 *Total British Sickness and Invalidity Benefit for incapacities has increased between 1955 and 1993*

Individuals with disc prolapse commonly present with minor sensory disturbances and with alteration of the reflexes in the lower limbs. These are not specific indications for referral, but do help in establishing the exact diagnosis.

The patients usually present with back pain and occasionally with sciatic scoliosis. Straight-leg raising is usually restricted with a positive sciatic stretch test on straight leg raising, with pain felt in the calf and the ankle or foot.

If conservative treatment is not successful then percutaneous treatment with chemonucleolysis is successful in 70% of cases, discectomy and decompression of the nerve root is successful in 80–90% of cases. Occasionally where symptoms are mild or the patient is not suitable for surgery an epidural may resolve the symptoms in about one in three patients.

Sciatica is usually a self-limiting disease, and treatment is mainly helpful to accelerate recovery. This is particularly true of sciatica caused by disc prolapse. Surgery should only be considered where there is significant neurological dysfunction, or where pain is not resolving at 6 weeks.

Scoliosis

Scoliosis usually presents in childhood. Occasionally elderly ladies do present with a degenerative type of scoliosis which may give rise to symptoms of spinal instability or even spinal stenosis.

Scoliosis is a relatively common condition, with 10% of children having a slight scoliosis. A scoliosis requiring surgery is only present in two in 1000 children. The three main types are neurogenic scoliosis, congenital scoliosis of a structural type, and the most common in this country, idiopathic scoliosis. Neurogenic and structural type scoliosis usually present relatively early in life, and an early referral for a specialist opinion is indicated. Idiopathic scoliosis may present early (10% of cases), but the vast majority (90%) present during the adolescent years as adolescent idiopathic scoliosis. These patients need to be reassured, providing there is no obvious underlying cause for the scoliosis, that it is simply a cosmetic condition.

Any child with a significant scoliosis should be referred for a specialist opinion.

Spinal stenosis

This condition typically presents in individuals over 60 years of age. It is usually associated with degenerative changes in the lumbar spine, and a combination of loss of disc space, new bone formation due to osteophytes and infolding at the ligamentum flavum initially compress the nerve roots laterally but ultimately may cause a central type of stenosis. At worst, this may cause symptoms of cauda equina compression. The symptoms are usually of insidious onset, and increasing gradually over a number of years. There is not usually any associated injury. Fifty per cent of patients will present with significant back pain, and most patients will have a history of back pain. The typical symptoms are of pain in the leg with or without weakness or numbness, which usually occurs on walking. The patients are typically better walking up hill than down hill,

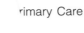
**ive clinical features of spinal stenosis, peripheral vascular
ease**

	Spinal stenosis	Disc prolapse	Peripheral vascular disease
ͻ.ιι leg raise	Sometimes	Yes	No
..ͻgical deficit	Sometimes	Yes	No
Leg pain on walking	Yes	Sometimes	Yes
Leg pain on sitting	No	Yes	No
Pain relief on standing still	No	No	Yes
Pain relief on sitting	Yes	No	Yes
Numbness/paraesthesiae	Yes	Yes	No

Emergency and urgent referrals

The initial diagnostic triage will identify the small number of patients requiring urgent and emergency referral to a hospital specialist. Guidelines for emergency and urgent referrals are set out below.

Emergency referral:

Diagnosis:	Acute spinal cord damage/acute cauda equina syndrome/widespread neurological disorder.
Action:	Emergency referral to a specialist with experience in spinal surgery within a matter of hours.

Urgent referrals (within a few weeks):

Diagnosis:	Possible serious spinal pathology.
Action:	Urgent referral for specialist investigation, generally to an orthopaedic surgeon or a rheumatologist, depending on local availability.

Diagnosis:	Possible acute inflammatory disorders.
Action:	Urgent referral to a rheumatologist.

Diagnosis:	Nerve root problem.
Action:	Should generally be dealt with initially by the GP, providing there is no major progressive motor weakness. Early referral may be required for additional acute pain control. If it is not resolving satisfactorily after 6 weeks, the patient should therefore be referred urgently for appropriate specialist assessment and investigation.

Fig. 5.11 *Indications for emergency and urgent referral. (Adapted from Clinical Standards Advisory Group, 1994)*

and are better cycling than walking, as flexion of the spine tends to have the effect of decompressing nerve roots to some extent. Occasionally the patient will present with bowel or urinary symptoms but again the symptoms are generally of rather gradual onset.

Physiotherapy is not particularly helpful for this condition. Approximately 30% of individuals will achieve some relief of their symptoms, especially if they have some back pain, with the use of a lumbar corset. Epidurals are occasionally indicated although the success rate is probably only about 20%. Epidural injections may be difficult due to the narrow epidural space. Calcitonin injections given four times a week for 4 weeks have been shown to be helpful in about 25% of patients with this condition. However, the injections usually only give relative relief of the symptoms, although occasionally symptoms do resolve completely. General practitioners may be asked to supervise the prescription and injection of the calcitonin. Side-effects include nausea and hot flushes.

Surgery is indicated in patients who have not responded to conservative measures. Only patients with significant symptoms, either affecting their day-to-day life or preventing them working, will be considered for surgery. The initial success rates for this type of surgery are approximately 70%.

Spinal infection

Spinal infection is rare and patients present with a constant unremitting back pain, particularly at night. The pain often keeps them awake. They may complain of rigors or a temperature. Spasm is often present in the paraspinal muscles and patients are usually tender at the site of the infection, although clinical signs are notoriously unreliable. This condition is common in individuals with immunological disorders such as diabetes, and also in individuals who have had cardiac or urinary catheterization. Urgent referral is indicated, as early treatment with intravenous antibiotics is usually successful.

Spinal tumours

Ninety per cent of spinal tumours are due to secondary tumour, and therefore a majority of the patients presenting with this will have a history of a previous malignant tumour. Like infection, the symptoms are usually of gradually increasing pain which is constant in nature, and may keep the patient awake at night. There may be neurological signs if there is compression on the spinal cord or the nerve roots. Plain X-ray is useful in assisting diagnosis, but early referral is recommended. Most of these patients will respond to radiotherapy, but occasionally surgery is necessary either for compressive symptoms or rarely for an unresolved pain.

Imaging techniques

Indications for X-ray

X-rays are of limited value in the diagnosis and management of the majority of patients with spinal disorders. They are not usually indicated in the initial management of acute back pain in patients between 20 and 55 years. It has been estimated that approximately 1% of X-rays change the management of patients. X-rays may be of value in diagnosis in some cases of mechanical disorder, such as spondylolisthesis.

X-rays may be of value in the diagnosis of spinal infection, metastases and spinal tumours but MRI is more sensitive in diagnosis and is of more value.

Plain X-rays are of no value in the diagnosis of disorders such as disc prolapse and spinal stenosis.

Other imaging techniques

In the future MRI may be available by direct access for general practitioners.

Interpretation of the results of MRI scanning is difficult. For example, it has been demonstrated that up to 20% of individuals will have asymptomatic disc prolapses, and that nearly 100% of individuals will have degenerate discs by the age of 70.

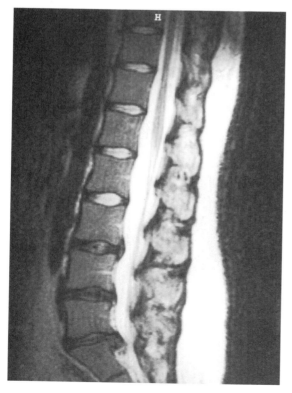

Fig. 5.12 *MRI showing a prolapsed L5/S1 disc*

Case Histories

1

A young man presents with a foot drop and sciatica of 1 week's duration.

Appropriate management includes:

Simple analgesics	1
NSAIDs	1
Rest	1
Physiotherapy	0
Use of splints/support/bandage	0
Aspiration	0
Steroid injection	0
Blood test	0
X-ray	0
Routine referral	0
Urgent referral	1
Emergency referral	0
None of these	0

Surgeon's view: This is an acute disc prolapse with neurological loss. Pain relief and urgent referral are indicated.

2

A woman of 45 presents with bad back pain for 3 weeks preventing her sleeping at all at night, with pain at rest during the day.
You might manage her with:

Simple analgesics	1
NSAIDs	1
Rest	0
Physiotherapy	0
Use of splints/support/bandage	0
Aspiration	0
Steroid injection	0
Blood test	1
X-ray	1
Routine referral	0
Urgent referral	0
Emergency referral	1
None of these	0

Surgeon's view: This is an alarming presentation and infection or tumour must be excluded. Emergency referral is indicated.

3

A 33-year-old car factory worker has been unable to work for 3 weeks because of acute back pain. He has no sciatica.

Appropriate management would be:

Simple analgesics	1
NSAIDs	1
Rest	1
Physiotherapy	1
Use of splints/support/bandage	0
Aspiration	0
Steroid inject	0
Blood test	0
X-ray	0
Routine referral	0
Urgent referral	0
Emergency referral	0
None of these	0

Surgeon's view: Acute back pain. Rest and analgesia is the treatment of choice.

4

A 45-year-old cleaner presents with chronic back pain of 9 months' duration. The pain is related to activity and she has been unable to work for 4 months. There are no real features of a depressive illness.

Suitable management might include:

Simple analgesics	1
NSAIDs	1
Rest	0
Physiotherapy	1
Use of splints/support/bandage	0
Aspiration	0
Steroid injection	0
Blood test	0
X-ray	0
Routine referral	0
Urgent referral	0
Emergency referral	0
None of these	0

Surgeon's view: This woman has mechanical low back pain. She will probably respond to treatment with analgesia and physiotherapy.

5

A 70-year-old man presents with back pain and sciatic symptoms. His leg pain prevents him from walking more than 200 yards. Physiotherapy has not been helpful.

Which of the following would be appropriate:

Simple analgesics	1
NSAIDs	1
Rest	0
Physiotherapy	1
Use of splints/support/bandage	0
Aspiration	0
Steroid injection	0
Blood test	0
X-ray	1
Routine referral	1
Urgent referral	0
Emergency referral	0
None of these	0

Surgeon's view: This man has symptoms of spinal stenosis and he may benefit from surgery. Routine referral is indicated.

6

A 40-year-old lady presents with sciatica of 3 days' duration with a depressed ankle jerk and loss of sensation in S1.

Which of the following might be useful in her management:

Simple analgesics	1
NSAIDs	1
Rest	1
Physiotherapy	1
Use of splints/support/bandage	0
Aspiration	0
Steroid injection	0
Blood test	0
X-ray	0
Routine referral	0
Urgent referral	0
Emergency referral	0
None of these	0

Surgeon's view: These symptoms are probably due to disc prolapse. They will almost certainly respond to analgesia and rest.

7

A 23-stone (146 kg) lady presents with bilateral sciatica and straight-leg raising of 20 degrees normal power and reflexes in the legs, and frequency of micturition. She has no perineal sensation.

Appropriate management would be:

Simple analgesics	0
NSAIDs	0
Rest	0
Physiotherapy	0
Use of splints/support/bandage	0
Aspiration	0
Steroid injection	0
Blood test	0
X-ray	0
Routine referral	0
Urgent referral	0
Emergency referral	1
None of these	0

Surgeon's view: The most likely diagnosis is a central disc prolapse and emergency referral should be made.

8

A 45-year-old manual worker has had mechanical back pain for 2 years. He was seen and fully assessed a year ago in the orthopaedic clinic and discharged. He has been off work for 9 months and physiotherapy and treatment by a chiropractor were not helpful.

Appropriate management would be:

Simple analgesics	1
NSAIDs	1
Rest	0
Physiotherapy	0
Use of splints/support/bandage	1
Aspiration	0
Steroid injection	0
Blood test	0
X-ray	0
Routine referral	1
Urgent referral	0
Emergency referral	0
None of these	0

Surgeon's view: Mechanical low back pain with failure to respond to appropriate conservative measures. Referral should be made for consideration of fusion.

9

A 14-year-old girl presents with a scoliosis and back pain of 1 month's duration and has been off school for 2 weeks.

Appropriate management might include:

Simple analgesics	1
NSAIDs	1
Rest	0
Physiotherapy	1
Use of splints/support/bandage	0
Aspiration	0
Steroid injection	0
Blood test	1
X-ray	1
Routine referral	0
Urgent referral	1
Emergency referral	0
None of these	0

Surgeon's view: An acute painful scoliosis in this age group requires urgent investigation to exclude infection, tumour and progression of her scoliosis.

10

Your patient underwent discectomy at L4/5 2 years ago. She has been thoroughly investigated, but no cause has been found for her persistent postoperative sciatica and she has been discharged. She returns finding this sciatica intolerable.

Appropriate management includes:

Simple analgesics	1
NSAIDs	1
Rest	0
Physiotherapy	1
Use of splints/support/bandage	0
Aspiration	0
Steroid injection	0
Blood test	0
X-ray	0

Routine referral   1
Urgent referral   0
Emergency referral   0
None of these   0

Surgeon's view: Routine referral is indication to consider management of her pain.

Further reading

Spitzer, W. O. et al. (1987). Scientific Approach to the Assessment and Management of activity-related spinal disorders. A monograph for clinicians. Report of the Quebec Task Force on Spinal Disorders. *Spine*, **12**; S1.

Benn, R. T. and Wood, P. H. N. (1975). Pain in the back. An attempt to estimate the size of the problem. *Rheumatol. Rehabil.*, **14**; 121.

Powell, M. C. et al. (1986). Prevalence of lumbar disc degeneration observed by magnetic resonance in symptomless women. *Lancet*, **ii**; 1366 (8520).

Hakelius, A. (1970). Prognosis in sciatica. A clinical follow-up of surgical and non-surgical treatment. *Acta Orthop. Scand. (Suppl.)*, **129**; 1.

Clinical Standards Advisory Group (1994). *Back Pain*. HMSO, London.

6

Hip
Richard de Steiger

- Referral for hip replacement surgery should be based on individual disability and levels of pain – old age is not a contraindication.
- Loosening of the hip joint replacement occurs in 5% of patients at 10 years.
- Trochanteric bursitis responds well to steroid injections.
- Septic arthritis of the hip may present insidiously.

Presenting symptoms

Adult hip problems invariably present with pain in the groin and thigh. Symptoms may radiate to the knee.

Stiffness and leg shortening may also be a feature, particularly in arthritis, and will usually cause an abnormal gait. A limp is a common feature of hip pathology.

Physical examination

Hip examination should include a brief assessment of gait though abnormalities may only be apparent if the patient has walked for some distance. An antalgic gait is one in which the patient, because of pain, spends less time on the affected side during the stance phase of gait leg length should be checked, especially to note if there is any apparent discrepancy because of fixed hip deformity. A passive range of motion is next carried out and often internal rotation is the first movement lost. A normal range of motion for a hip joint is 120 degrees of flexion, 40 degrees of abduction, 30 degrees of adduction, 40 degrees of external rotation and 30 degrees of internal rotation. As lumbar spine problems can commonly present as pain around the hip joint, examination of the lumbar spine and, if appropriate, a lower limb neurological examination must be performed.

Table 6.1 Common causes of hip pain in different age groups

Age group	Cause Intra-articular	Periarticular	Referred
Childhood (2–10 years)	Developmental dislocation of the hip Perthe's disease Irritable hip Rickets	Osteomyelitis	Abdominal
Adolescence (10–18 years)	Slipped upper femoral epiphysis Torn labrum	Trochanteric bursitis Snapping hip Osteomyelitis Tumours	Abdominal Lumbar spine
Early adulthood (18–30 years)	Inflammatory arthritis Torn labrum	Bursitis	Abdominal Lumbar spine
Adulthood (30–50 years)	Osteoarthritis Inflammatory arthritis Osteonecrosis Transient osteoporosis	Bursitis	Abdominal Lumbar spine
Old age (>50 years)	Osteoarthritis Inflammatory arthritis		Abdominal Lumbar spine

Table 6.2 Normal range of movement: hip

Flexion	0–120 degrees
Extension	0–30 degrees
Abduction	0–45 degrees
Adduction	0–30 degrees
Internal rotation	0–45 degrees
External rotation	0–45 degrees

Common hip problems

Arthritis

Almost any cause of systemic arthritis can involve the hip joint, but by far the most common is osteoarthritis (OA). Radiographic signs of hip OA may affect between 5 and 10% of the population to a varying degree and although small joints are most commonly affected in rheumatoid

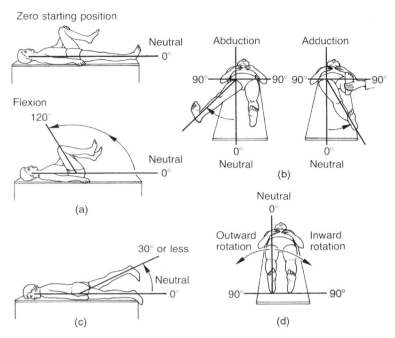

Zero starting position

Neutral 0°

Flexion 120°

Abduction 90° — 90°

Adduction 90° — 90°

Neutral 0°

0° Neutral (b)

(a)

30° or less

Neutral 0°

(c)

Neutral 0°

Outward rotation — Inward rotation

90° — 90°

(d)

Fig. 6.1 *a, Flexion; b, abduction/adduction; c, extension; d, rotation*

Table 6.3 Indications for hip replacement surgery

Pain	This is the principal indication for surgery. Pain that occurs at rest and at night, severe pain on movement and pain poorly controlled with analgesic medication are also strong indicators
Activities of daily living	If the restricted movement and pain caused by the arthritis are significantly affecting ability to walk, dress, wash, etc. then this is a relative indication for total hip replacement
Age	Because joint replacements have a limited survival, surgery under the age of 55 or 60 has to be considered especially carefully

arthritis, the hip is involved as the disease progresses. The various inflammatory arthropathies and other metabolic disorders may all involve the hip.

The early clinical symptoms of hip arthritis are manifested by dull groin pain radiating to the buttock, lateral thigh and often to the knee. The

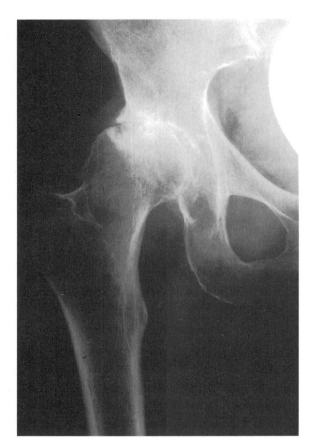

Fig. 6.2 *X-ray of an osteoarthritic hip*

pain is exacerbated by movement, in particular standing from a seated position, and is worse at the end of a long day. Rest improves the pain, but, as the disorder progresses, rest and nocturnal pain become significant. The earliest clinical examination features are loss of internal rotation and this is followed by reduced flexion and abduction. Patients begin to limp, especially after walking for a distance, and commonly complain that they are unable to perform simple tasks such as putting on shoes and socks or having a bath. The back should also be examined as patients with OA have an increased incidence of degenerative lumbar spine disease. Classic X-ray of findings of OA are joint space narrowing, osteophytes, subchondral sclerosis and cyst formation, and these are present in varying degrees according to the severity.

Management of this widespread condition is based on treating the patient's main symptom, which is pain, and the secondary symptom, which is disability. Patients initially need some education about the natural history of OA as many think they are doomed to a progressive downhill course, leaving them severely disabled. This is not the case, and the symptoms from hip OA tend to wax and wane and do not always irretrievably worsen.

Many people wish to know what they can and cannot do in terms of daily activities and sporting pursuits. As a general rule, the more vigorous and demanding a sport the more likely the patient is to suffer from hip pain during or after the event. The patients can be instructed to be sensible about pursuing activities and there is certainly no reason for them to stop. Activities such as walking, swimming, bicycle riding and gardening can all be continued without undue risk to the hip. If the patient knows that a particular activity is likely to cause pain, then it is sensible for them to take analgesics prior to them undertaking the activity.

For the pain, simple analgesics are the first line of therapy. There is little good evidence that NSAIDs alter the course of osteoarthritis. Though they may provide some initial pain relief, they do not have a role in long-term management. Maintaining a range of movement in any arthritic joint is important, and simple exercises, swimming and, in more severe cases, a referral to a physiotherapist for hydrotherapy treatment are of value.

A stick, used in the contralateral hand, will help unload the force through the affected joint and improve gait. A simple shoe insole may also help some people. Weight loss is recommended and will certainly be beneficial if surgery is required, but is in practice difficult to achieve and unlikely to help the patient's symptoms significantly.

The decision to refer for surgical therapy is based largely on the level of the pain and the disabilities the patients suffer. Loss of independence, particularly in elderly people, and an inability to work in younger people are other facts to be taken into account. Intracapsular hip joint injection may have some limited therapeutic value, but can be diagnostic if there is doubt as to whether the pain is lumbar or hip related. Total joint replacement has revolutionized the treatment of hip osteoarthritis, but osteotomy and, in some cases, arthrodesis of the hip should still be considered in the younger patient. Following hip replacement patients usually require 7–10 days' stay in hospital and are discharged on crutches or a stick.

As a result of the large number of primary hip replacements performed, many artificial joints are now becoming loose, resulting in the need for revision hip replacement. This is an increasing problem and as a general rule any patient that has recurrence of pain in a previously replaced joint should be sent for specialist advice. Plain X-rays are often difficult to interpret.

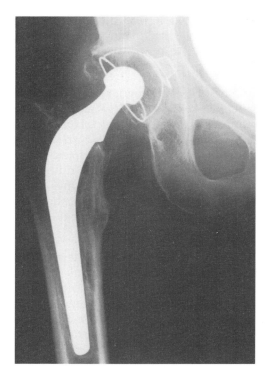

Fig. 6.3 *X-ray of a total hip replacement*

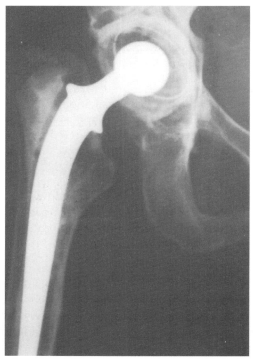

Fig. 6.4 *X-ray of a loose total hip replacement*

Table 6.4 Indications of problems with a hip replacement

Pain	Any significant and sustained increase in pain around a joint replacement should be investigated. If in doubt refer. Some patients have a persistent ache around the hip and thigh, even in an otherwise succesful joint replacement
Loss of movement	Artificial joints are often stiff but a sudden loss of movement should be investigated with a radiograph
Leg-length discrepancy	Some patients will have leg-length discrepancy from the outset, this can usually be corrected with a heel raise
Dislocation	Occasionally hip replacements dislocate, this is invariably a painful and acute event and requires emergency referral. The leg will usually appear short and externally rotated
Fracture	Fractures can occur around artificial joints, particularly if they are loose. They usually present acutely with severe pain and loss of function. Emergency referral is indicated
Loosening	Aseptic loosening of joint replacements occurs in about 5% of cases at 10 years. It will usually present with gradual onset of pain and should be investigated with an X-ray. If loosening is present then refer
Infection	Deep infection is rare after joint replacements (<3%). It will usually present with pain. Sometimes local signs are present. Rarely the patient may be systemically unwell, emergency referral is indicated in these situations
DVT and pulmonary embolus	DVT is common after lower limb joint replacement. Isolated calf vein thromboses can be treated conservatively but thrombi extending higher than the knee are probably best treated with heparin and 3 months warfarin. Deaths from pulmonary emboli are rare (<1%)

Avascular necrosis

Avascular necrosis (AVN), or osteonecrosis, is a disorder which may affect several bones, but does commonly present in the hip joints. As the name implies, there is an interruption to the blood supply of the femoral head which classically results in a pathological, crescent-shaped fracture of the femoral head. Patients at risk of developing this condition include immuno-suppressed patients with renal transplants, patients receiving steroid therapy, patients who have sickle cell disease, deep-sea divers and patients who have a high alcohol intake. The commonest cause, however, is a delayed presentation following trauma to the femoral head or neck. Typically the patient presents with a dull pain in the groin which is usually exacerbated by weightbearing. The condition is frequently bilateral in the non-traumatic group but presenting at different time periods. X-rays may be entirely normal in the early stages, but usually when a patient is sympto-matic, they reveal a subchondral fracture of the femoral head. MRI will show medullary changes of AVN before any radiographic changes.

Referral is appropriate early and the outcome is largely dependent on the amount of involvement of the femoral head. Many treatments have been proposed for AVN of the hip which may relieve pain, but do not always alter the long-term outcome. In the early stages of AVN, core decompression by drilling a hole up through the femoral neck may relieve pain. In several centres, bone grafts are inserted into the femoral head with the aim of revascularizing the dead bone. This has shown some promising results. Osteotomy to replace an area of dead bone with a viable articular cartilage may be performed in selected cases.

Acetabular dysplasia

Acetabular dysplasia is a condition in which the acetabulum fails to fully develop and at maturity is shallow, leaving the anterolateral part of the femoral head uncovered. People, more frequently females, usually present in their third to fourth decade with hip pain after exercise, or a busy day. This usually disappears with rest but can persist. Examination of the hip reveals a full range of movement which is usually irritable only in the extremes of flexion and internal rotation. Sometimes patients who have an acetabular labral tear complain of a feeling of instability, in which case examination of the hip in extension and external rotation reproduces this feeling of instability.

X-rays reveal a shallow acetabulum with femoral head subluxation of a varying degree and early arthrosis may be present. This condition, if left untreated, may lead to increasing pain and eventually arthritis of the hip joint, especially if there is an incongruity between the femoral head and the acetabulum.

Referral is indicated to discuss the natural history of the disorder and to plan treatment options. To relieve symptoms and prevent the onset of arthritis some form of cover of the femoral head is required. This can be achieved by introducing a simple shelf of bone over the capsule or by more complex peri-acetabular osteotomies. Unfortunately, in some instances the joint is incongruent and this leads to secondary OA and the need for joint replacement.

Infection

Although this is a relatively uncommon problem in the adult hip, it is important to diagnose because failure to do so and treat may have disastrous effects on the hip joint itself. Septic arthritis of the hip is more common in childhood but over the last few decades there has been an increasing incidence in adults. Bacteria can infect the hip joint, generally through three mechanisms: haematogenous spread, spread from a nearby focus, or direct inoculation at the time of a procedure or trauma. As with other forms of infection, certain patients are at risk, including those with chronic diseases, such as diabetes, renal failure, rheumatoid arthritis, immunocompromised patients, especially if on systemic steroids, and patients who are malnourished. The commonest organisms involved are *Staphylococcus aureus* and streptococcus. Tuberculosis, however, must always be considered. The onset may sometimes be insidious, but pain is the presenting feature and the patient may complain of fever and chills. Patients may not always be febrile but the hip is extremely irritable on examination and sometimes cannot be moved.

Referral for treatment is a matter of urgency, and diagnosis can be made on ultrasound-guided aspiration or athrotomy. Specimens of tissue should be sent for gram stain and microscopy immediately. Treatment is formal washout of the joint, followed by appropriate intravenous antibiotics, according to the microbiological diagnosis. If treatment is prompt the joint can usually be salvaged, but, in longstanding cases, cartilage destruction and secondary OA may result.

Tumour

Primary bone tumours affecting the hip area are rare, but metastatic spread of tumour to the proximal femur and acetabulum are much more commonly encountered. Carcinoma of the breast, colon, prostate and thyroid, amongst other neoplasms, may all metastasize to the hip. Sometimes, in fact, the presenting symptom for an undiagnosed primary is pain around the hip.

In any patient undergoing treatment for carcinoma who presents with vague deep-seated pain, metastatic bone spread should always be considered. Plain films will usually show up any significant lesions but a bone scan is more sensitive in detecting smaller tumours. Patients should be treated surgically if severe pain cannot be controlled or the bone is in imminent danger of fracture. Cemented joint replacement or hemiarthroplasty may provide relief from pain and give a patient mobility. Operations are indicated even though the patient's life span is shortened. The patients are at slightly higher risk of wound breakdown from deep infection in this instance, especially if there has been prior radiotherapy to the involved area.

When treating a young adult for a presumed soft tissue problem around the hip which does not improve or worsens, beware of deep, continuous pain, especially if unrelated to activity and occurring nocturnally. Osteosarcoma, though rare, must be born in mind and investigated by X-ray.

Soft tissue problems about the hip

Underlying muscle strains and tendonitis

Muscle strains about the hip can occur from sudden violent exercise, whilst tendonitis usually occurs from repetitive chronic overuse. Common sites involved around the hip are the ischial tuberosity at the origin of the hamstring muscles and along the edge of the pubic ramus at the origin of the adductor longus. The pain is usually localized to these specific areas but may radiate down the thigh. With acute trauma cold packs and compression to restrict bleeding are indicated. In the more chronic conditions non-steroidal anti-inflammatory medication, heat and ultrasound all have a role to play. Injection at the tender site with local anaesthetic and cortisone is reserved for resistant cases.

Trochanteric bursitis

This condition is an inflammation of the bursa over the greater trochanter. It is most commonly seen in runners. Patients complain of a deep aching, located on or just behind the greater trochanter, and often are unable to sleep on the affected side. There is well-localized tenderness to palpation over the trochanter. This is usually a self-limiting condition and can be treated initially with heat and topical non-steroidal creams. If the condition persists, a local anaesthetic and steroid injection into the most tender spot will usually resolve the symptoms. This is a safe procedure to perform using 40 mg of steroid preparation and 2–5 ml of marcaine.

Snapping hip syndrome

This is a condition, usually found in dancers and adolescent girls, whereby the iliotibial band rubs or snaps over the greater trochanter. The patients complain of a click or snap when they flex and rotate their hip, although the condition occurs intermittently and is uncomfortable rather than painful. Usually treatment is reassurance that nothing seriously is wrong, and most patients ignore the symptom. Occasionally, in some people with persistent or painful symptoms, lengthening the iliotibial band is indicated.

Case Histories

1

A 32-year-old man who had a renal transplant peformed 2 years ago presents with vague pain in the groin. The pain is not related to exercise.

Simple analgesics	1
NSAIDs	1
Rest	1
Physiotherapy	0
Blood test	0
X-ray	1
Steroid injection	0
Routine referral	1
Urgent referral	0
Emergency referral	0
None of these	0

Surgeon's view: Because the patient is young and is probably on immunosupressant therapy, avascular necrosis of the hip should be suspected. Simple analgesics and rest may help the pain and an X-ray may well be normal. If the pain persists referral is indicated.

2

A 55-year-old man with a long history of alcohol abuse and smoking presents with a 3-day history of feeling generally unwell. He states that he has had pain in his groin which is becoming more severe, and on examination the hip is extremely painful.

Simple analgesics	1
NSAIDs	0
Rest	0
Physiotherapy	0
Blood test	1
X-ray	1
Steroid injection	0
Routine referral	0
Urgent referral	0
Emergency referral	1
None of these	0

Surgeon's view: Septic arthritis is one of the few true emergencies in orthopaedic surgery and must be suspected in any patient who has an extremely painful joint with no prior history of disease or trauma. Emergency referral is indicated and blood tests, X-rays and ultrasound should be performed. This is best done at a specialist centre.

3

A 27-year-old mother of two small children presents with pain in the groin radiating into the lateral aspect of the hip joint. She states that she has had this intermittently for several years but has noticed that things have become worse now that she is looking after two active children. The pain is always much worse at the end of the day and tends to resolve overnight.

Simple analgesics	1
NSAIDs	1
Rest	1
Physiotherapy	0
Blood test	0
X-ray	1
Steroid injection	0
Routine referral	1
Urgent referral	0
Emergency referral	0
None of these	0

Surgeon's view: This lady gives a good story of fatigue pain in the hip which may be soft tissue related or related to acetabular dysplasia. If simple analgesics and NSAIDs fail to help the pain then an X-ray should be performed. If dysplasia is present referral to a specialist hip clinic is indicated.

4

A 50-year-old lady with a past history of a mastectomy presents with sudden severe pain in the right groin radiating down the anterior aspect of the thigh. This came on while she was getting out of bed in the morning. She is barely able to walk and examination reveals that the right hip is painful on all ranges of movement.

Simple analgesics	0
NSAIDs	0
Rest	0
Physiotherapy	0
Blood test	0
X-ray	1
Steroid injection	0
Routine referral	0
Urgent referral	0
Emergency referral	1
None of these	0

Surgeon's view: This lady is likely to have suffered a pathological fracture in the hip joint from breast metastases. Emergency referral is indicated for fixation or joint replacement as indicated.

5

A 92-year-old man who lives with his wife in a small cottage presents with severe pain in both hips. He is now unable to sleep without regular codeine analgesics and he depends on home help daily. His wife confides to you that she finds it more and more difficult to cope and is worried that he may have to go into a home.

Simple analgesics	1
NSAIDs	1
Rest	1
Physiotherapy	0
Blood test	0
X-ray	1
Steroid injection	0
Routine referral	1
Urgent referral	0
Emergency referral	0
None of these	0

Surgeon's view: This man is likely to have bilateral hip arthritis which has been impossible to control with medical therapy. Despite his age, if his general health is good he will benefit from joint replacement.

6

A 20-year-old man who regularly plays football at the weekends presents with a 6-month history of groin pain. He feels that it started when he was kicked across the leg during a football match and notices that at the end of every Saturday the pain is worse. It settles down overnight but is interfering with his training.

Simple analgesics	1
NSAIDs	1
Rest	1
Physiotherapy	1
Blood test	0
X-ray	1
Steroid injection	1
Routine referral	1
Urgent referral	0

Emergency referral   0
None of these   0

Surgeon's view: This young man is likely to have chronic adductor strain of his hip joint. If NSAIDs and physiotherapy do not work, then a steroid/local anaesthetic injection into the affected area may be beneficial.

Injection of lateral aspect of the hip

Indications

For trochanteris bursitis.

Technique

With the patient laying on the side palpate the greater trochanter. The point of maximum tenderness is usually just posterosuperior to the trochanter. Insert an 18-gauge needle and inject at a depth of 2–3 cm over a wide area.

Usually use 5 ml of a combination of **either** 10–25 mg hydrocortisone acetate, **or** 5–10 mg triamcinalone, **or** 10–20 mg methylprednisolone with 1% lidocaine.

Frequency

Every 4–6 weeks. If there is no benefit after two or three injections then consider alternative treatment or referral.

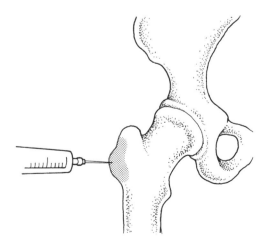

Fig. 6.5 *Injection of lateral aspect of the hip*

Structures at risk

Injection directly onto bone or periosteum is exquisitely painful, so try and avoid it.

Further reading

Balderston, R. A., Rothman, B. W., Booth, R. E. and Hozack W. J. (1992). *The Hip.* Lea and Febiger, Philadelphia.

Steinberg, M. E. ed. (1991). *The Hip and its Disorders.* W. B. Saunders, Philadelphia.

7

Knee _____ Christopher A. Dodd

- Anterior knee pain in adolescents is common and treatment is conservative.
- X-ray examination of the knee is rarely helpful in the younger patient.
- Degenerative meniscal tears characteristically cause nocturnal knee pain.
- Anterior cruciate rupture is the most common knee injury caused whilst skiing.
- Steroid injections into the knee should be intra-articular

Presenting symptoms

Assessment of the presenting symptoms should differentiate between the symptoms detailed below.

Pain

Whether it is localized (and therefore highly significant) or diffuse (and less likely to signify surgical pathology).

Swelling

Whether it occurs immediately after an injury, suggesting a haemarthrosis as seen in a cruciate rupture, or whether it develops overnight, implying a reactive effusion such as occurs with a meniscal tear.

Locking

This term often causes confusion. Locking is specifically a recent inability to fully extend the knee, implying a mechanical block such as a torn meniscus.

Clicking/catching

Usually described when ascending/descending stairs and suggests patellofemoral articular cartilage damage.

Table 7.1 Common causes of knee pain in different age groups

Age group	Cause		
	Intra-articular	Periarticular	Referred
Childhood (2–10 years)	Juvenile arthritis Osteochondritis dissecans Infection Torn discoid meniscus	Osteomyelitis	Perthes' disease Irritable hip
Adolescence (10–18 years)	Osteochondritis dissecans Torn meniscus Anterior knee pain syndrome Patellar maltracking	Osgood–Schlatter's disease Sinding–Larsen–Johnson syndrome Osteomyelitis Tumours	Slipped upper femoral epiphysis
Early adulthood (18–30 years)	Torn meniscus Instability Anterior knee pain syndrome Inflammatory arthritis	Ligament injuries Bursitis	
Adulthood (30–50 years)	Degenerate meniscal tears Osteoarthritis Inflammatory arthritis	Bursitis	Osteoarthritis of hip
Old age (>50 years)	Osteoarthritis Inflammatory arthritis	Bursitis	Osteoarthritis of hip

Anterior aspect
patella and patellar ligament are turned upwards
femur at 90° to tibia   Posterior aspect

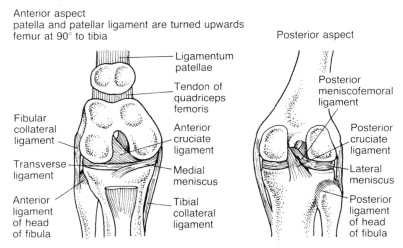

Fig. 7.1 *Ligaments around the knee*

Giving way

Is a mechanical event which occurs when the weightbearing knee in slight flexion is put under sudden extra stress such as in running and 'cutting' to the side. This is the hallmark symptom of a cruciate ligament rupture.

Physical examination

Look

Physical examination should begin with an inspection of the knee, with the patient standing upright. The degree of overall alignment from in front (varus/valgus) and from the side (hyperextension/flexion deformity) should be measured. Quadriceps wasting occurs quickly with disuse, and is best assessed by comparing active contraction and noting vastus medialis obliquus muscle bulk.

The presence of swellings around the knee should be noted. Localized swellings suggest extra-articular pathology, whereas intra-articular swelling is seen above and to the side of the patella.

Previous scars, signs of a recent injury, and infection should be documented, particularly looking for areas of bruising, discoloration and swelling.

Palpate

Palpation can often be useful particularly if there is local tenderness, suggesting focal pathology, rather than diffuse tenderness which suggests generalized inflammation. A large, tense swelling indicates a haemarthrosis or a pyarthrosis, whereas a lax swelling is usually secondary to an effusion associated with synovitis.

The presence of an effusion is assessed by stroking the fluid from the suprapatellar pouch distally. Any evidence of synovial thickening should be noted. **A clinically obvious effusion is always significant**. A popliteal swelling or cyst may be palpated at the back of the knee and is usually more prominent in extension.

Move

Examination of the movement of the joint should begin by lifting both heels. Sagittal deformity (fixed flexion/hyperextension) will become obvious. A 'springy block' to full extension suggests significant meniscal pathology, whereas a solid block usually suggests longstanding pathology such as osteoarthrosis.

The active, followed by the passive, range of movement should then be documented. Range of motion is then assessed, looking in particular for loss of motion and for how smoothly the movement takes place. The extensor mechanism should be palpated and, in particular, any irritability and/or crepitus noted. The patient should be assessed sitting on the edge of the couch actively flexing and extending the knee. With a hand on the patella any lateral subluxation will be obvious.

Table 7.2 Normal range of movement: knee

Flexion	0–135 degrees

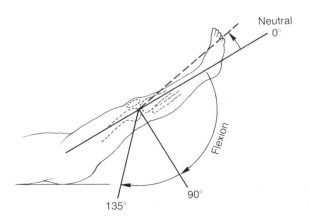

Fig. 7.2 *Flexion and extension*

Specific tests should then be undertaken:

McMurray: Internal/external rotation of the flexed knee, looking for pain and clicking over the medial/lateral jointline (assessment of posterior horn meniscal pathology).

Lachman: Attempted anterior drawer of the tibia on the femur in 20 degrees flexion (most sensitive test for anterior cruciate damage).

Anterior drawer (Figure 7.3): As Lachman, but attempted at 90 degrees flexion (less specific test). With the knee flexed to 90 degrees and the hamstrings relaxed, attempt to draw the tibia forwards. In anterior cruciate deficiency there will be excessive movement.

Finally, examination of the knee should conclude with an assessment of the hip joint above and of the spine to exclude referred pain. Examination should include an assessment of the neurology of the lower limb.

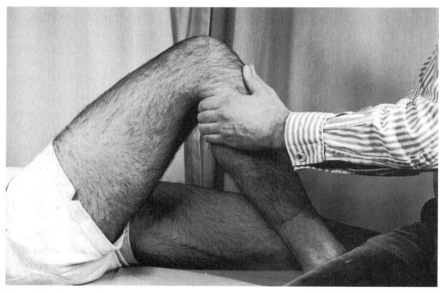

Fig. 7.3 *Testing for knee instability – the anterior draw test*

Common knee problems

Discoid meniscus

This presents in young patients (2–10 years old), and may be bilateral with clicking, catching usually of the lateral joint line and chronic symptomatology. Examination may reveal minor flexion contracture with joint line tenderness. Investigation with radiographs may reveal a widened joint space. An MRI scan is usually diagnostic. If the knee is symptomatic, then an arthroscopic examination may be indicated. Menisectomy is usually only undertaken if the meniscus is torn.

Anterior knee pain syndrome

This syndrome usually affects adolescents, girls much more commonly than boys, with spontaneous onset, bilateral distribution and recurrence. Often the history of symptoms goes back 1 or 2 years. Pain is often aggravated by climbing stairs, changing gears in a car, prolonged sitting and wearing high heels. Examination will often reveal retropatellar crepitus and irritability. Quadriceps weakness may be present and the hamstrings are sometimes tight, otherwise examination is remarkably unremarkable. Investigation with radiographs is usually worthless and not indicated. MRI is normally reserved as a last resort after failed physiotherapy treatment and for reassurance. Conservative treatment is advised. This is generally a self-limiting problem. Detailed explanation and reassurance is required. NSAIDs and splintage in the acute phase can be helpful. Bracing may be added as the patient improves. Physiotherapy is very important, and the patient may need repeat sessions. Surgery is very limited, and is contemplated only after failure of prolonged conservative treatment. Arthroscopy is performed to exclude other causes. Sometimes a lateral release is advised, but this procedure is not without complications. Major bony surgery is also unpredictable. Patellectomy can be undertaken but it may not be curative and is associated with a large number of early and late complications.

Patellar malalignment

This is common in adolescence, particularly girls. Patella alta, genu valgum, external tibial torsion and persistent femoral anteversion are all causes of this problem. Acute dislocation may be associated with osteochondral fracture. Patellar subluxation is much more common than dislocation. On examination there may be very little to see. Look for quadriceps wasting and patellar irritability with and without crepitus. The apprehension sign (apprehension as the examiner attempts to laterally displace the patella) and medial retinacular tenderness in the acute case are particularly significant. Plain radiographs, including a skyline view, are useful in the assessment of patellar tilt and/or subluxation. MRI scanning with 'dynamic' views of the patella tracking offers promise in the assessment of these patients and may well be able to predict which patients may require surgery. Conservative treatment is usually advised, including exercises and bracing. Surgery for the failed conservative group remains controversial. Arthroscopic lateral release is popular but not without complications and this procedure has less than a 60% success rate. Tibial tubercle transfer is probably more predictable but is significantly more invasive.

Meniscal tear

This usually occurs in the young adult with a sports-related injury (e.g. soccer). Twisting on the weightbearing leg is a common history. The patient may complain of clicking, catching and locking if they are suffering from a big tear. Meniscal tears are often associated with an anterior cruciate injury (ACL) injury. The younger patient usually presents with a longitudinal or parrot-beak variety of tear, whereas the older patient presents with a horizontal or radial tear (degenerate variety). On examination quadriceps muscle wasting is almost an invariable finding. A joint effusion (delayed onset) with joint line tenderness and a positive McMurray's test with or without a clunk should be actively looked for. A minor flexion deformity with a springy block to extension (if large displaced tear) is very significant. Radiographs are rarely helpful, but an MRI is useful if doubt exists about the diagnosis. Arthroscopic meniscectomy is the treatment of choice. Longitudinal, peripheral tears are repaired if possible.

Anterior cruciate rupture

This affects the young adult involved in a sports-related injury. Usually the trauma is as a result of a non-contact injury with the patient falling to the floor. Immediate swelling is a very common presentation. The patient may describe a pop or crack. The pain is usually intense and the injured person is often taken to casualty. Acute symptoms last a week or so, then settle. Once the acute phase is over the patient often complains of recurrent giving way, saying the knee 'feels unstable' on returning to sports. Examination is often difficult immediately after the injury but a haemarthrosis may be present. A positive Lachman test is invariably present (AP draw at 20 degrees) whereas a positive anterior draw (AP draw at 90 degrees) may be difficult to elicit because of pain and spasm. There may be signs of a positive pivot shift test, indicating anterolateral rotatory instability. Signs of meniscal damage should also be sought by examining for joint line tenderness and a positive McMurray's test. Radiographs may be useful acutely to exclude bony injury in the very painful presentation, otherwise they are rarely helpful. MRI is very useful for assessing both cruciate ligament and meniscal damage. Conservative treatment includes proprioceptive hamstring rehabilitation and allows the acute injury to settle. Reconstruction is appropriate for younger sports patients or those patients who have functional symptoms despite conservative treatment.

Degenerative meniscal tear

This is seen in middle-aged patients with a fairly innocuous injury. Indeed they may not remember a traumatic episode. Chronic symptomatology with night pain is highly specific. Twisting manoeuvres tend to exacerbate symptoms. Quadriceps wasting with a minor flexion deformity and joint line tenderness is very suggestive of significant 'surgical' pathology. X-ray may reveal minor osteoarthritis.

MRI reveals the characteristic appearance of a tear. Arthroscopic partial meniscectomy is the treatment of choice if there are major signs of mechanical disruption or if a steroid injection fails to settle symptoms.

Symptomatic loose body formation

This is a relatively rare presenting complaint. Episodes of sudden severe pain/swelling should raise the possibility of this condition, with the joint being reasonably symptom free in between acute episodes. Quadriceps wasting with a minor flexion deformity and an effusion are usual. A palpable loose body (usually suprapatellar pouch) confirms the diagnosis. X-rays are diagnostic if a true loose body is seen. The intercondylar view is often particularly useful. Few reported 'loose bodies' are in fact **loose**.

Arthroscopic assessment and surgery with removal of the loose body is the usual outcome.

Early osteoarthritis

This is seen in middle-aged patients sometimes with a previous injury. Pain/swelling with activity is usual. Pain is usually improved with rest. NSAIDs frequently help greatly. Quadriceps wasting and diffuse joint line tenderness with a minor flexion contracture usually indicate degenerative pathology.

Physiotherapy is very likely to be of major benefit in the early case. Intra-articular steroid injection is frequently useful in the recurrent case and arthroscopy is reserved for those cases that fail to settle with the aforementioned measures.

Established osteoarthritis

This presents in middle to old age with chronic symptoms. Acute exacerbations usually settle quickly. There is pain/swelling with activity. Established flexion and varus/valgus deformity with reduced movement are sometimes present. Irritability, crepitus with movement and often secondary ligamentous laxity is encountered. A weightbearing X-ray is usually very helpful, a standard lateral less so. For patellofemoral OA, a skyline view is helpful. MRI is not usually helpful.

NSAIDs, physiotherapy, weight reduction, walking stick, etc. should be tried in the first instance. Bracing the knee is often helpful if instability is a problem. Arthroscopic surgery is unpredictable, but can give dramatic relief. The role of arthroscopic abrasion chondroplasty is yet to be defined, but usually helps with mechanical symptoms.

Bursitis

Bursitis is a common problem due to inflammation of the bursae around the knee.

Prepatellar bursitis (housemaid's knee)

This is an occupational hazard in people who spend a great deal of time kneeling, such as carpet-layers, etc.

There is a hot, tender well-circumscribed, fluctuant lesion over the front of the patella, which may look infected but usually is not.

Most lesions settle with rest and avoidance of kneeling. Occasionally aspiration is necessary which often has to be repeated. If this fails then surgical excision is occasionally required.

Infrapatellar bursitis (clergyman's knee)

This fits the description of prepatellar bursitis, with the swelling below the patella over the tendon.

Tendonitis

This presents with pain with or without swelling of the tendons around the knee, usually associated with overuse.

Patellar tendonitis (jumper's knee)

This most commonly affects young sportsmen. Symptoms are related to the inferior pole of the patella and are exacerbated by activity, particularly climbing stairs, running and jumping. Pain and swelling over the inferior pole of the patella are often present.

Most cases respond to rest and NSAIDs. In persistent cases an injection of steroid/anaesthetic is usually curative.

Other relatively common sites of tendonitis around the knee are:

1. Iliotibial band friction syndrome (runner's/cyclist's knee).
2. Hamstring tendonitis.
3. Medial ligament syndrome.
4. Popliteus sydrome.

Osteochondritis dissecans

This is seen in boys much more than girls, with the second decade being the usual presentation, but it may occur earlier. Pain with activity and clicking or giving way may occur.

There is mild effusion usually with quadriceps wasting and tenderness over the site of the lesion (medial femoral condyle). Locking occurs if the fragment separates, with a loose body usually felt in the supra-patellar pouch. X-rays are usually diagnostic and tunnel views the most helpful.

MRI/bone scan is occasionally needed. An undisplaced fragment in the younger child is treated with rest. Loose fragments are replaced and fixed if possible or excised in the chronic case.

Osgood–Schlatter disease

This is traction apophysitis of the tibial tuberosity. It is seen in children of 10–14 years most commonly and is associated with overuse. There is pain with or without enlargement of the tuberosity.

X-ray usually shows characteristic fragmentation of the tuberosity.

The symptoms usually settle with rest. Surgical excision of the fragments is rarely necessary.

Sindig–Larsen–Johansson syndrome

This is analogous to Osgood–Schlatters disease, occurring at the distal pole of the patella.

Chondromalacia patellae

This literally means softening of the articular cartilage but this diagnosis can only be made at arthroscopy. This should not be used as a generic term as it is a pathological term. It may be associated with anterior knee pain syndrome and patella maltracking.

The idiopathic variety usually responds to the conservative measures of isometric quadriceps exercises with or without bracing.

Bipartite patella

This problem is usually seen as a lucent line at the superolateral corner of the patella and can be mistaken for a fracture. It occurs when the ossification centres of the patella fail to fuse. Surgery is rarely required.

Plica syndrome

This is often diagnosed but is rarely a specific cause of knee pain. It is caused by failure of the breakdown of the embryonic synovial shelves which normally occurs by the fourth intrauterine month. Medial plica is most often implicated and diagnosis is suspected by palpating a tender thickened band over the medial femoral condyle.

Steroid injection should be tried, followed by arthroscopic resection if this fails.

Septic arthritis and osteomyelitis

This is a relatively common disorder with infection, usually blood borne from the upper respiratory tract. The patient presents with severe pain and a tense effusion. The slightest movement causes agony and the patient is usually unwell.

Appropriate antibiotics should be commenced immediately and arthro-scopic washout instigated as an emergency. Arthrotomy is required if the pus has loculated. The differential diagnosis includes other inflam-matory pathologies, including non-specific synovitis and Still's disease.

Acute haematogenous osteomyelitis commonly affects the proximal tibial/distal femoral metaphyses. The patient is usually unwell with local tenderness and a high WBC/CRP/ESR.

Popliteal cysts and swellings (Baker's cyst)

This is a common finding which can occur at any age. Most cysts communicate with the knee joint and the semimembranosus bursa on the medial side of the knee is most often implicated.

There is swelling with or without pain at the back of the knee, which is usually more prominent when the knee is extended. There may be restricted flexion. In children there is often no other abnormality but in the older patient intra-articular pathology is the norm.

Differential diagnosis includes popliteal artery aneurysm and tumours. MRI is usually the investigation of choice.

In children most regress with time. In the adult treatment should be directed at the underlying cause. Surgical excision is rarely required and the recurrence rate is high.

Synovial pathology

Recurrent effusions of spontaneous onset, with or without pain, can occur. Patients present with diffuse swelling/thickening, mainly felt above the patella, usually with quadriceps wasting and a mild flexion deformity.

Non-specific synovitis

This is a relatively common problem, of spontaneous onset, which occurs mainly in early adulthood. Patient may relate recent non-specific illness.

Inflammatory blood screen is routine. This may settle with rest but a steroid injection may be required. Recurrent symptoms which fail with conservative treatment require arthroscopic synovectomy where histology shows non-specific features. Occasionally the condition may progress to an inflammatory picture such as rheumatoid arthritis. Surgery is usually curative.

Pigmented villonodular synovitis

This condition occurs in young adults and is characterized by a proliferative synovial reaction. The aetiology is unknown and the knee joint is the most common site of presentation. Mechanical symptoms are common and pain is invariable. Arthroscopic synovectomy is the modern treatment of choice, but this may need to be repeated.

Synovial chrondromatosis

This is a rare condition of unknown aetiology, secondary to metaplasia in the subsynovial connective tissue with pedunculated or loose cartilagenous bodies within/around the knee joint. It usually occurs in middle age and the patient presents with pain and swelling. Examination reveals synovial thickening with palpable loose bodies. Synovectomy and loose body removal is usually successful at alleviating the majority of the patient's symptoms.

Table 7.3 Indications for knee replacement surgery

Pain	This is the principal indication for surgery. Pain that occurs at rest and at night, severe pain on movement and pain poorly controlled with analgesic medication are also strong indicators
Activities of daily living	If the restricted movement and pain caused by the arthritis are significantly affecting ability to walk, dress, wash, etc., then this is a relative indication for knee replacement
Age	Because joint replacements have a limited survival, surgery under the age of 55 or 60 has to be considered especially carefully

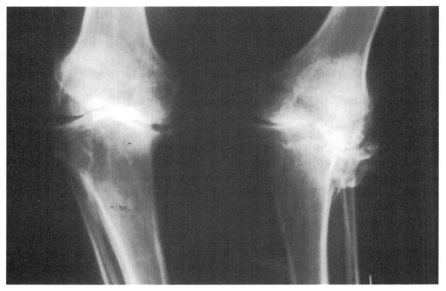

Fig. 7.4 *X-ray showing osteoarthritis of the knee*

Table 7.4 Indications of problems with a knee replacement

Pain	Any significant and sustained increase in pain around a joint replacement should be investigated. If in doubt refer. Some patients have a persistent ache around the hip and thigh, even in an otherwise succesful joint replacement
Loss of movement	Artificial joints are often stiff but a sudden loss of movement should be investigated with a radiograph
Fracture	Fractures can occur around artificial joints, particularly if they are loose. They usually present acutely with severe pain and loss of function. Emergency referral is indicated
Loosening	Aseptic loosening of joint replacements occurs in about 5% of cases at 10 years. It will usually present with gradual onset of pain and should be investigated with an X-ray. If loosening is present then refer
Infection	Deep infection is rare after joint replacements (<3%). It will usually present with pain. Sometimes local signs are present. Rarely the patient may be systemically unwell, emergency referral is indicated in these situations
DVT and pulmonary embolus	DVT is common after lower limb joint replacement. Isolated calf vein thromboses can be treated conservatively but thrombi extending higher than the knee are probably best treated with heparin and 3 months warfarin. Deaths from pulmonary emboli are rare (<1%)

Magnetic resonance imaging (MRI)

The MRI scan can be invaluable but its exact role requires definition.

It is very sensitive/specific for meniscal/ligamentous injuries but its resolution for articular cartilage damage is, as yet, poor.

Presently it is used mainly in anterior knee pain to exclude a surgical lesion and as a diagnostic aid in unexplained knee pain.

In general it provides about 70% of the information obtained by arthroscopy.

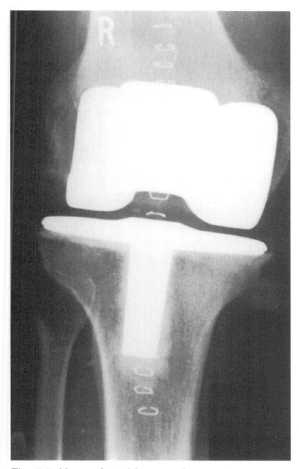

Fig. 7.5 *X-ray of total knee replacement*

Case Histories

1

A 12-year-old girl presents with clicking and intermittent pain in the left knee. Examination reveals locking and lateral joint line tenderness.

Simple analgesics	1
NSAIDs	0
Rest	1
Physiotherapy	0
Splints/support/bandages	0
Aspiration	0
Steroid injection	0
Blood test	0
X-ray	0
Routine referral	1
Urgent referral	0
Emergency referral	0
None of these	0

Surgeon's view: A discoid lateral meniscus is likely, and if pain and symptoms persit referral is appropriate.

2

A 12-year-old boy presents with spontaneous onset of pain in his knee for the past 3 months. Examination reveals generalized tenderness otherwise normal.

Simple analgesics	1
NSAIDs	0
Rest	1
Physiotherapy	0
Splints/support/bandages	1
Aspiration	0
Steroid injection	0
Blood test	0
X-ray	0
Routine referral	0
Urgent referral	0
Emergency referral	0
None of these	0

Surgeon's view: Anterior knee pain is the most probable diagnosis. Rest and support bandages and reassurance are most appropriate.

3

A 16-year-old girl presents with a 2-year history of knee pain exacerbated by running and descending stairs. Examination reveals minor quadriceps wasting and lack of terminal extension of the knee.

Simple analgesics	1
NSAIDs	1
Rest	0
Physiotherapy	1
Splints/support/bandages	0
Aspiration	0
Steroid injection	0
Blood test	0
X-ray	0
Routine referral	0
Urgent referral	0
Emergency referral	0
None of these	0

Surgeon's view: Chondromalacia or anterior knee pain are the likely diagnosis. Physiotherapy and NSAIDs are the most appropriate treatment.

4

A 17-year-old boy presents with a year's history of recurrent episodes of giving way of the knee. Examination reveals quadriceps wasting but no real tenderness. There is crepitus anteriorly with flexion.

Simple analgesics	1
NSAIDs	0
Rest	1
Physiotherapy	0
Splints/support/bandages	0
Aspiration	0
Steroid injection	0
Blood test	0
X-ray	1
Routine referral	1
Urgent referral	0
Emergency referral	0
None of these	0

Surgeon's view: Osteochondritis dissecans is likely and an X-ray should be arranged.

5

A 17-year-old boy presents with acute pain and swelling in the knee following a tackle during a game of football. Examination reveals generalized tenderness with painful movements otherwise normal.

Simple analgesics	1
NSAIDs	1
Rest	1
Physiotherapy	0
Splints/support/bandages	1
Aspiration	0
Steroid injection	0
Blood test	0
X-ray	0
Routine referral	0
Urgent referral	0
Emergency referral	0
None of these	0

Surgeon's view: A ligament sprain or meniscal injury are possible. Rest and analgesia should be advised. Only if symptoms persist is referral necessary.

6

A 17-year-old boy presents with acute pain and swelling in the knee following a tackle during a game of football. Examination reveals joint line tenderness, an effusion and the joint is locked.

Simple analgesics	1
NSAIDs	1
Rest	1
Physiotherapy	0
Splints/support/bandages	0
Aspiration	1
Steroid injection	0
Blood test	0
X-ray	0
Routine referral	0
Urgent referral	1
Emergency referral	0
None of these	0

Surgeon's view: A Meniscal injury is likely and an urgent referral is indicated. Aspiration of a tense effusion may produce symptomatic relief.

7

A 26-year-old girl presents with a 6-month history of recurrent, painless effusions in the knee. Examination reveals quadriceps wasting, an effusion and there is flexion deformity.

Simple analgesics	1
NSAIDs	1
Rest	1
Physiotherapy	1
Splints/support/bandages	1
Aspiration	0
Steroid injection	1
Blood test	1
X-ray	0
Routine referral	1
Urgent referral	0
Emergency referral	0
None of these	0

Surgeon's view: Synovitis is possible and physiotherapy and referral are indicated. Steroid injection and anti-inflammatory medication may also benefit.

8

A 29-year-old footballer injured his knee 1 year ago. On returning to the game his knee repeatedly gives way.

Simple analgesics	0
NSAIDs	0
Rest	0
Physiotherapy	1
Splints/support/bandages	1
Aspiration	0
Steroid injection	0
Blood test	0
X-ray	0
Routine referral	1
Urgent referral	0
Emergency referral	0
None of these	0

Surgeon's view: An anterior cruciate ligament injury is likely and physiotherapy and routine referral are indicated.

9

A 44-year-old man presents with recurrent pain and swelling over the medial aspect of his knee. Examination reveals an effusion and medial joint line tenderness.

Simple analgesics	1
NSAIDs	1
Rest	0
Physiotherapy	1
Splints/support/bandages	1
Aspiration	1
Steroid injection	1
Blood test	0
X-ray	1
Routine referral	1
Urgent referral	0
Emergency referral	0
None of these	0

Surgeon's view: Early osteoarthritis is likely and analgesics may help. If symptoms persist, then referral for physiotherapy and possibly arthroscopy are indicated. Steroid injection may also be of value.

10

A 50-year-old woman presents with recurrent pain and swelling within her knee. Examination reveals diffuse swelling and generalized tenderness.

Simple analgesics	1
NSAIDs	1
Rest	1
Physiotherapy	0
Splints/support/bandages	1
Aspiration	1
Steroid injection	1
Blood test	1
X-ray	1
Routine referral	1
Urgent referral	0
Emergency referral	0
None of these	0

Surgeon's view: Synovitis and arthritis are most likely. Rest and NSAIDs may help. If these measures fail, then an X-ray and referral are appropriate.

Lateral and medial injection of the knee

Indications

For arthritis of the knee and for other intra-articular causes of pain.

Technique

With the patient supine and the leg relaxed palpate and move it from side to side.

Insert an 18-gauge needle just at the level of the superior pole of the patella in the coronal plane. Aim to pass the needle to its full depth between the patella and the femur. Inject slowly into the joint. If an effusion is present then withdrawing on the syringe will confirm that you are in the joint.

Usually use 5 ml of a combination of **either** 25–50 mg hydrocortisone acetate, **or** 20 mg triamcinalone, **or** 40 mg methylprednisolone with 1% lidocaine.

Frequency

Every 4–6 weeks. If there is no benefit after two or three injections then consider alternative treatment or referral.

Structures at risk

Injection directly onto bone or periosteum is exquisitely painful, so try and avoid it.

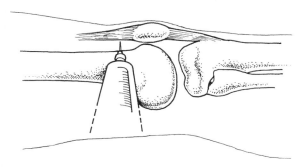

Fig. 7.6 *Lateral or medial injection of the knee*

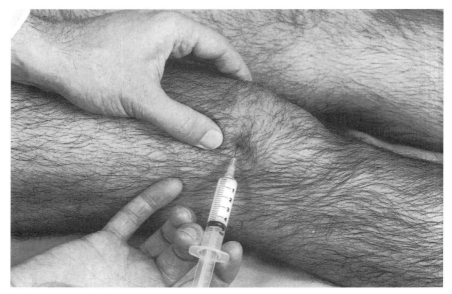

Fig. 7.7 *Lateral injection of the knee*

Anterior injection of the knee

Indications

For arthritis of the knee and for other intra-articular causes of pain.

Technique

With the patient supine and the leg relaxed and flexed to 90 degrees, palpate the patella tendon.

Insert an 18-gauge needle just lateral to the tendon and aim for the inter-condylar notch. Aim to pass the needle to its full depth. Inject slowly into the joint. If an effusion is present then withdrawing on the syringe will confirm that you are in the joint.

Usually use 5 ml of a combination of **either** 25–50 mg hydrocortisone acetate, **or** 20 mg triamcinalone, **or** 40 mg methylprednisolone with 1% lidocaine.

Frequency

Every 4–6 weeks. If there is no benefit after two or three injections then consider alternative treatment or referral.

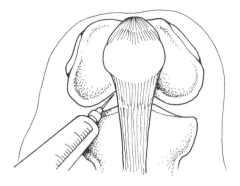

Fig. 7.8 *Anterior injection of the knee*

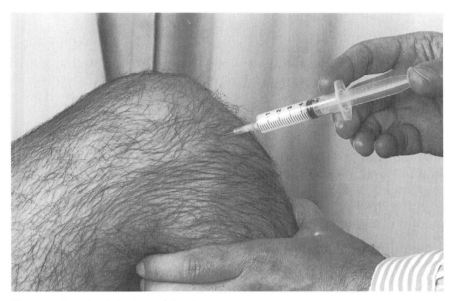

Fig. 7.9 *Anterior injection of the knee*

Structures at risk

Injection directly onto bone or periosteum is exquisitely painful, so try and avoid it.

8

Foot and ankle
Paul H. Cooke

- Many foot problems can be treated by restoring anatomical alignment.
- Collapse of the medial arch is a common cause of hindfoot and midfoot pain.
- Calcaneal spurs are rarely of clinical significance.
- Forefoot surgery is a major procedure – recovery may take up to 6 months.
- Steroids should not be injected into the Achilles tendon.

Presenting symptoms

The adult foot is a complex structure, with joints allowing flexion and extension at the ankle, inversion and eversion at the subtalar joint, rotation at the midtarsal region, and fine movements of the toes. The interaction of the joints means that often problems in different parts of the feet are functionally and causally related. This, coupled with a complex language used to describe foot problems, has led to a mystique, and often to a belief, that problems of the foot must be dealt with by a specialist of one sort or another.

In fact, many problems can be solved simply if certain principles are followed. The principles are based on the observation that the 'normal' healthy foot functions well in practice, and that many foot problems can be treated by restoring anatomical alignment.

Corns, callosities and other such painful lesions only occur due to abnormal pressure from within or outside the foot.

These principles should be remembered when addressing problems in the foot.

Common foot and ankle conditions

Hindfoot and midfoot pain

The common cause of pain in the hindfoot and midfoot is valgus hindfoot and collapse of the medial arch, which occur in middle age and

Table 8.1 Common causes of foot and ankle pain in different age groups

Age group	Cause Intra-articular	Periarticular	Referred
Childhood (2–10 years)	Club foot Congenital midfoot and forefoot deformities Septic arthritis	Osteomyelitis	
Adolescence (10–18 years)	Arch disorders (pes cavus pes planus)	Osteomyelitis Tumours	
Early adulthood (18–30 years)	Metatarsalgia Hallux valgus Hallux rigidus Osteochondritis Accessory ossicles	Achilles tendonitis Achilles tendon rupture Fasciitis	Lumbar spine Knee
Adulthood (30–50 years)	Osteoarthritis Inflammatory arthritis Gout Metatarsalgia Hallux valgus Hallux rigidus Osteochondritis Accessory ossicles	Ischaemic foot pain Diabetes Bursitis Tendonitis Plantar fasciitis Corns	Lumbar spine Knee
Old age (>50 years)	Osteoarthritis Inflammatory arthritis Gout Metatarsalgia Hallux valgus Hallux rigidus	Ischaemic foot pain Diabetes Bursitis Tendonitis Plantar fasciitis Corns	Lumbar spine Knee

beyond. The conditions are related, and one leads to the other if untreated. Both occur secondary to progressive weakness of the calf muscles.

The patient presents with foot pain which increases on walking, and which may restrict walking distance.

Assessment should be made of the position and angulation of the hindfoot and midfoot when standing.

The patient is observed from behind, and a visual line dropped vertically from the centre of the knee joint. This should pass through the centre of the ankle joint (and Achilles tendon) and to the centre of the

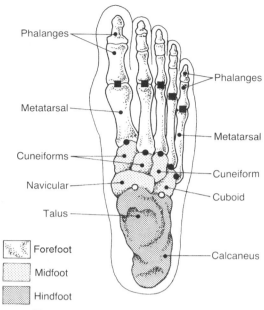

Phalanges

Phalanges

Metatarsal

Metatarsal

Cuneiforms

Cuneiform

Navicular

Cuboid

Talus

Calcaneus

Forefoot

Midfoot

Hindfoot

■ Metatarsophalangeal joints

● Tarsometatarsal joints

○ Midtarsal joint

Fig. 8.1 *Bone joints and regions of the foot*

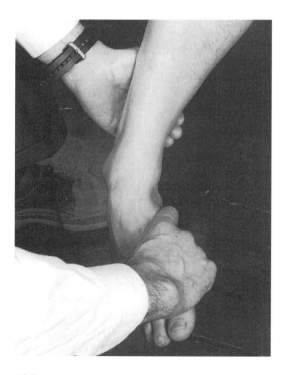

Fig. 8.2 *Testing for ankle instability*

heel. Commonly, when the hindfoot is painful, the ankle/subtalar joint is in valgus, and the line passes lateral to the ankle joint. If deformity is observed, test to see whether this is passively correctible with the patient sitting.

Next the patient should turn round, to face the examiner, and the arch of the foot should be observed. The patient should be asked whether the arch has 'dropped' compared with their normal stance. The arch should be observed with the heels on the ground, and then on standing on tiptoes. The mobility of the arch is thus assessed.

Treatment depends on whether the pain is due to valgus collapse of the hindfoot, collapse of the arch or both.

The objective of treatment is to position the foot beneath the leg, with the sole flat to the floor, and to strengthen the weak muscles.

Method 1: If the subtalar joint is not deformed, but the arch has dropped, supply an arch support. (Many shoes contain an arch support or a proprietary 'medial arch support' may be added.)

Method 2: If the subtalar joint is valgus, then the heel needs supporting in a vertical position. If the deformity is minor then it may again be corrected by a medial arch support which will force the heel straight. For more severe deformity the heel must also be directly supported. This may be acheived by supplying custom splints (extended heel cups – extended to include an arch support), or by wearing running trainers, as these shoes incorporate a firm heel counter and a firm medial arch support.

Whichever of these methods is adopted, the patient must be taught foot and calf exercises, or the relief and support from the orthoses will be short-lived.

Painful heel

Painful heel, plantar fasciitis or policeman's heel most commonly occurs in men in their fifties or sixties. It is characterized by pain beneath the heel which is worse on standing and which can often be pinpointed with accuracy.

The pain seems to arise from excess tension at the insertion of the plantar fascia into the calcaneum, again probably secondary to weakness of the intrinsic muscles of the calf and foot which allow the arch to sag creating excess tension in the plantar fascia.

On examination no abnormality can be detected other than a severely painful area beneath the heel. X-ray will often show a calcaneal spur, but only because it is such a common finding anyway. X-ray should generally be avoided unless there are atypical features, as patients often become fixated on a visible spur which is of no clinical significance.

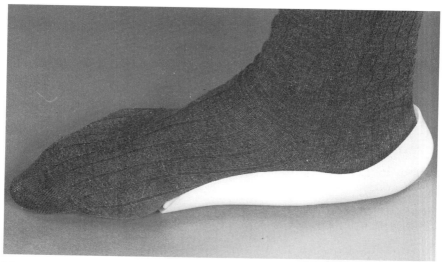

Fig. 8.3 *Heel cup for valgus heel deformity*

Treatment of mild cases comprises anti-inflammatory medication and physiotherapy with foot and calf exercises and local ultrasound. On occasions palliation may be obtained by wearing silicone heel pads or foam rubber heel pads. In more severe cases these can be trimmed centrally to give them the appearance of a horseshoe. In this instance the weight is carried completely away from the tender area.

Some cases are severe and do not respond to simple local treatment. In this case treatment is by injection of the painful area with local anaesthetic and steroid. This is an effective treatment but is itself painful. Few patients will wish to have the injection repeated and for this reason a long-acting depot-steroid should be used.

The natural history of this condition is that it rarely, if ever, lasts longer than 18 months or 2 years, provided surgical treatment is not undertaken. The outcome of surgical treatment is poor and the results of the release of the plantar fascia can be long-term painful flat foot, the consequences of which extend far beyond 2 years. For this reason referral is usually only worthwhile for provision of orthoses, or for further injection to be administered under anaesthetic.

Forefoot problems

Bunions

Bunions are a common condition in Caucasian races in whom they are often transmitted in families by autosomal dominant inheritance with variable penetrance. Patients present with symptoms relating to rubbing of the bunion on shoes or with concern about the natural history and progression of bunions, wanting treatment before they 'get as bad as granny's'.

Patients presenting with a bunion should be examined as described for hindfoot and midfoot pain. Both heel valgus and flat foot make bunions worse and on occasions cause them.

In cases with flat foot or valgus heel, correction of the medial arch will often correct the hallux valgus, reduce the width of the forefoot and ease the pain from the bunion.

To demonstrate whether an arch support will be effective the patient is made to stand with a small roll of foam beneath the medial arch or alternatively stand with the examiner's fingers held beneath and supporting the medial arch. The degree of correction can thus be demonstrated. If correction is obtained then a medial arch support should be advised. If it is not, and symptoms are severe enough to warrant surgical treatment, then the patient should be referred for a specialist opinion. Patients should be aware that forefoot surgery is a major, and on occasions painful, undertaking. Most operations require plaster or splintage for about 8 weeks, then a further 8 weeks until a shoe can be worn for a whole day. It is often 6 months or above before the foot has recovered to the preoperative level of function.

Table 8.2 Normal range of movement: forefoot

| Inversion | 0–35 degrees |
| Eversion | 0–15 degrees |

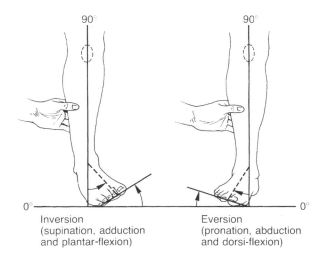

Inversion	Eversion
(supination, adduction	(pronation, abduction
and plantar-flexion)	and dorsi-flexion)

Fig. 8.4 *a, Inversion (supination, adduction and plantar-flexion); b, eversion (pronation, abduction and dorsi-flexion)*

Patients should not be referred because of worries about future progression of mild bunions, unless they can be seen to progress. It is not possible to predict future outcome, or to prevent severe bunions by early surgery. In any case, the variable penetration of the condition means that the severity of the condition will vary between generations.

Hallux rigidus

Hallux rigidus is a common painful condition of degenerative arthritis of the first metatarsophalangeal (MTP) joint, commonly occurring in the dominant foot of sports-orientated young men as they enter their twenties and thirties.

It causes pain particularly on kneeling with the toe tucked beneath the foot, and when crouching, running etc.

The diagnosis can be confirmed by palpation of the first MTP joint when a ridge of osteophyte will be felt circumferentially. Unlike the osteophyte palpable in hallux valgus (the bunion), the osteophyte of hallux rigidus can be felt on the dorsum and lateral side of the joint. The joint is always tender on palpation between the first and second ray. Similarly, dorsiflexion of the great toe is restricted and painful.

Symptomatic relief can be obtained by advising the patient to keep their toe straight when kneeling (and not to tuck it beneath the foot), or by stiffening the footwear. This may be done by selecting footwear with a rigid sole, by addition of a stiffening bar to the sole of the shoe or by insertion of a rigid insole.

If the patient continues to complain of symptoms or develops rest and night pain or pain which interferes with occupation, then surgical referral is advised. Surgery will often be similar to bunion surgery, and the same recovery period applies. In some centres arthroscopic surgery for minor cases is now becoming popular.

Metatarsalgia

Metatarsalgia is a condition in which pain is felt beneath the metatarsal heads. It may occur beneath a single metatarsal or beneath two or more metatarsals. Commonly it occurs in patients who have a relatively higher arch (a cavus foot).

The diagnosis is made on the symptoms, and the patient usually describes a feeling as though they are 'walking on a pebble'.

Examination of the foot may reveal a high arch and in more severe cases may reveal corns or calluses beneath the metatarsal heads. In severe cases and those associated with generalized arthropathies then ultimately dislocation of the MTP joints occurs.

Treatment is directed to relief of pain. In many cases, good relief can be obtained by trimming the calluses. If the relief obtained by such chiropody is longstanding, and particularly in elderly and unfit patients, then this may be all the treatment that is needed.

Additional relief may be obtained by the use of metatarsal pads. These can be obtained in two forms. The first is a pad with adhesive backing which is inserted into the shoe. The second is a pad on an elastic strap which is held beneath the foot by passing the elastic strapping around the forefoot.

Such pads are often sold with inadequate instructions, and it is important to advise the patient that the pad must be worn proximal to the area of pain so that the weight is transferred through the pad into the metatarsal neck. If, as commonly happens, it is worn beneath the corn or tender area then it will increase the problem.

The patient should be referred if they do not respond to local measures or pads.

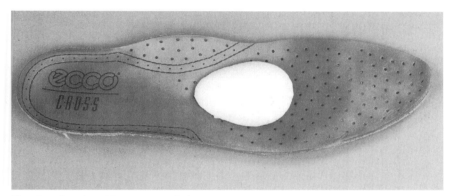

Fig. 8.5 *Insole with metatarsal dome*

Morton's neuroma

A small number of patients who have symptoms similar to metatarsalgia complain of severe lancinating pain which radiates down into the cleft between two toes and is associated with numbness of the adjoining skin of the two toes. This is caused by a benign inflammatory neuroma of the interdigital nerve (a Morton's neuroma).

This is diagnosed by compression of the metatarsals which causes pain and pain can also be induced by pressure on the sole of the foot in the interdigital area.

Neuromas can be treated by injection with local anaesthetic and steroid. The neuroma is palpated from the sole of the foot and the injection is made through the dorsum of the foot on to the identified point. The neuroma lies deep to the skin on the sole of the foot, so the injection needs to be deep into the foot.

If the pain fails to respond, or there is later remission, referral for a surgical opinion is required.

Toe deformities

Deformities of the lesser toes may be categorized and described as follows (Figure 8.6)

1 Curly toes – toes which curl into flexion but which are passively correctable.
2 Claw toes – curly toes which are uncorrectable.
3 Hammer toes – toes in which there is flexion of the proximal interphalangeal joint and extension of the distal interphalangeal joint.
4 Mallet toes – where there is flexion of the distal interphalangeal joint only.

Deformities of the toes are only important when they rub on the footwear (either the upper or the sole.)

Hammer toes frequently have corns on the dorsum of the proximal interphalangeal joint. Claw toes have callosities and corns over the dorsum of the proximal interphalangeal joint or beneath the tip of the toe (where the soft skin of the tip of the toe is directed into the sole of the shoe). Mallet toes have corns on the tip of the toe.

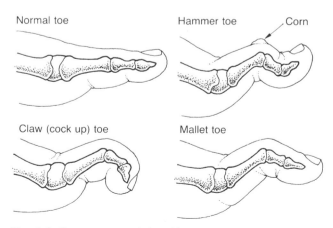

Fig. 8.6 *Common toe deformities*

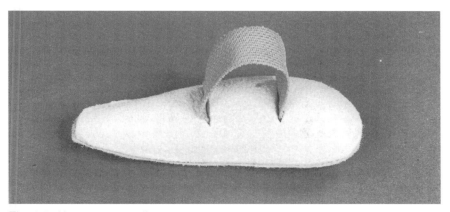

Fig. 8.7 *Hammer toe splint*

Treatment is always to relieve the pain, by protecting the painful area or by surgery.

Local chiropody may provide temporary relief when a hard corn rubs, but often it is the better and cheaper option to surgically correct the toes unless the patient is very frail. When long-term palliation is needed, or when problems arise only with certain footwear (e.g. walking boots), then corn pads may protect the skin.

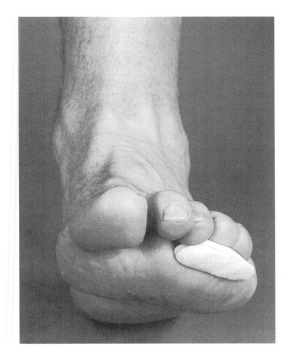

Fig. 8.8 *Banana splint for curly toes*

129

It may be appropriate to buy shoes with a high toe cap to prevent rubbing of the dorsum of the toe on the shoe, and/or to use a soft 'banana' splint (which tucks beneath curly or clawed toes), to elevate the tips of the toes from the sole of the shoe.

In fit patients who get substantial symptoms, referral for surgery is indicated to prevent long-term conservative treatment. Because the risk of infection in the toes is high, elderly patients who have joint replacements elsewhere in the body should also be referred, as surgery may prevent the chance of secondary infection.

Traditional fusion/correction of the toes requires a pin in the toes for 8 weeks which needs to be removed. More recently, techniques which avoid the use of pins have been developed and these reduce the high infection rate of pins and speed up recovery.

Ingrown toenails

Ingrown toenails are almost limited to the great toenail. They are predisposed to by flattening of the arch (when the great toe is rolled over), by pressure from ill-fitting shoes or by trauma. They often present with acute infection and granulation of long standing.

A history should be taken to find whether there are predisposing events such as a new pair of ill-fitting shoes or poor pedicure, and the foot should be examined for predisposing hindfoot and midfoot deformity. The nail should be observed end on and an assessment made of the curvature of the edge of the nail. Nails which substantially curl down at the edges are unlikely to respond to local treatment.

Local measures such as curettage of the nail, simple wedge resection, etc., may be tried with a reasonable prospect of success if a predisposing factor is identified and can be avoided in the future. Simple removal is indicated for a single episode of ingrown toenail in adolescence or adult, but there is no indication for undertaking recurrent simple removals.

If recurrences of ingrowing toenail occur, then removal with nail bed ablation should be performed. The choice as to whether this should be wedge resections or complete resections is a personal balance. The risk of recurrence is greater with wedge resections although the cosmesis is better.

Achilles tendon problems

Two conditions particularly affect the Achilles tendon, namely Achilles tendonitis and Achilles tendon rupture. It is believed that both are ruptures of fibres of the Achilles tendon. In the case of Achilles tendonitis, just one or two fibres rupture at a time, causing severe pain and inflammatory response.

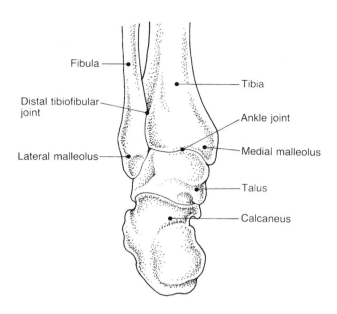

Fig. 8.9 *The bones of the ankle*

Fibula

Distal tibiofibular joint

Lateral malleolus

Tibia

Ankle joint

Medial malleolus

Talus

Calcaneus

Table 8.3 Normal range of movement: ankle

Plantarflexion	0–50 degrees
Dorisflexion	0–20 degrees

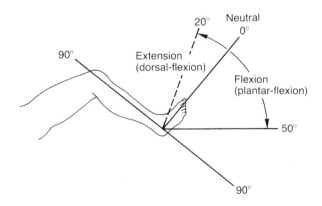

Fig. 8.10 *Extension and flexion*

Achilles tendonitis

The patient with Achilles tendonitis may be any age. Achilles tendonitis often arises after excessive use. Thus it may occur in younger people training for marathons or road running and equally may occur in the elderly. The patient presents with severe pain around the Achilles tendon which often increases on standing on tiptoes. There is usually a diffuse swelling around the Achilles tendon and it is always locally tender.

It is important to differentiate it from Achilles tendon rupture and this differential can be made by the squeeze or Thompson's test. The patient lies face down on the couch with their feet hanging over the end of the couch.

If the normal calf is squeezed firmly then the foot will plantarflex. In cases of rupture, squeezing the calf will lead to at most a tiny flicker of movement if the plantaris tendon remains intact.

Although there are other tests for Achilles tendon rupture, most of them can give false positives or false negatives and this is the definitive test.

Having made the diagnosis of Achilles tendonitis, then the patient should be treated by reducing their level of activities and with anti-inflammatory medication.

Many patients find it more comfortable to raise the heel slightly. They can often do this by putting on different shoes from their wardrobe, but for men and ladies who only have flat shoes then a cushioned heel insole such as that used for policeman's heel is often effective.

If these measures fail, then a period of 4 weeks in plaster of Paris almost always cures the problem.

Steroids should not be injected into the Achilles tendon, as this is often accompanied by tendon rupture (which is actually rare in the absence of steroid injections).

Referral to a specialist will be uncommon unless this is the only way to gain access to a plaster of Paris.

On occasions Achilles tendonitis is accompanied by a feeling of nodules where small ruptures have healed and calcified and these are sometimes referred because of suspicion of a tumour. Tumours of the tendo Achilles are vanishingly rare, and the diagnosis can be excluded unless there has been rapid growth of a lump beyond 2 cm.

Achilles tendon rupture

Achilles tendon rupture happens much more commonly in men, usually around their forties. However, it can affect a wide range of people. The commonest history is the feeling of a snap or being struck behind the heel often whilst playing badminton or squash. The patient often thinks their partner has hit them with a racquet and occasionally the partner attends, having been hit back with a racquet! Rupture can also occur as a consequence of other accidents and the commonest of these is missed footing on a step or ladder or breakage of a ladder rung. All these activities lead to forced sudden dorsiflexion of the foot.

The back of the heel is always tender and swollen. Thompson's test (as described above) is always positive, and this should always be performed and a note should be made of the results.

Although surgeons differ as to whether they should treat Achilles tendon ruptures conservatively or surgically, all would agree that they must be treated promptly and actively. Whether surgery is undertaken or not, the patient will need to be in plaster for 8–12 weeks after an Achilles tendon rupture.

Any patient with an Achilles tendon rupture should be referred urgently to hospital. The results of surgical treatment are heavily affected by the degree of the swelling and the state of the soft tissues, and for this reason it is important to elevate the leg as much as possible and if possible pack it with cold compresses/ice packs to reduce soft tissue damage whilst awaiting transfer.

In some series up to half of all Achilles tendon ruptures are missed and the possibility of a delayed presentation should be considered in any patient who has sprained their ankle and continues to limp. Again, a Thompson's test will be positive. However, there is a pitfall for the unwary. If the tendo Achilles itself is examined more than 3 months after the rupture then it will be felt to be intact. Unless a Thompson's test is performed, it may be assumed that the Achilles tendon did not rupture. In fact, what will have happened is that the tendon has ruptured and has healed in its lengthened state. Squeezing the calf will still lead to a negative result. The patient will be disabled and will have a permanent limp unless surgery is undertaken.

The decision as to whether to operate on a missed rupture becomes increasingly difficult as time passes from rupture to presentation. However, these patients do warrant urgent referral to an orthopaedic surgeon.

Case Histories

1

A 25-year-old man complains of pain in the great toe. On examination he has little or no bunion but pain and stiffness of movement of the great toe.

Simple analgesics	1
NSAIDs	1
Rest	0
Physiotherapy	0
Splints/support/bandage	1
Aspiration	0

Steroid injection	0
Blood test	0
X-ray	1
Routine referral	1
Urgent referral	0
Emergency referral	0
None of these	0

Surgeon's view: He has hallux rigidus. The diagnosis may be confirmed by X-ray. Most cases settle with analgesia and stiff shoes, but some require surgery. The alternative diagnosis of acute gout is usually obvious due to its sudden and severe nature.

2

A patient attends for a routine review, 1 year after a total hip replacement. She complains of a painful toe, and examination shows fixed clawing with ulceration over the proximal interphalangeal joint.

Simple analgesics	0
NSAIDs	0
Rest	0
Physiotherapy	0
Splints/support/bandage	1
Aspiration	0
Steroid injection	0
Blood test	0
X-ray	0
Routine referral	0
Urgent referral	1
Emergency referral	0
None of these	0

Surgeon's view: Any source of sepsis in a patient with a joint replacement must be treated seriously. If antibiotics and protective dressings/corn plasters do not lead to early resolution, she should be referred urgently for a surgical opinion, as she is at risk of secondary infection to her prosthetic joint whilst the source of sepsis remains.

3

A 45-year-old lady complains of pain beneath the second metatarsal and a feeling of 'walking on a pebble'.

| Simple analgesics | 0 |
| NSAIDs | 0 |

Rest	0
Physiotherapy	0
Splints/support/bandage	1
Aspiration	0
Steroid injection	0
Blood test	0
X-ray	0
Routine referral	1
Urgent referral	0
Emergency referral	0
None of these	0

Surgeon's view: Many cases of metatarsalgia will settle with simple orthotic measures. Surgery is often helpful if it does not.

4

A 58-year-old man complains of severe pain beneath his heel. On examination there is no abnormality other than local tenderness.

Simple analgesics	1
NSAIDs	1
Rest	1
Physiotherapy	1
Splints/support/bandage	1
Aspiration	0
Steroid injection	1
Blood test	0
X-ray	0
Routine referral	0
Urgent referral	0
Emergency referral	0
None of these	0

Surgeon's view: Policeman's heel is a self-limiting condition, but very painful. It should be treated actively and the patient should be reassured of the natural history.

5

A 70-year-old lady complains of severe ankle and hindfoot pain and 'going over' on her ankle. On examination from behind she has valgus deformity of the hindfoot.

Simple analgesics	1
NSAIDs	1

Rest	0
Physiotherapy	0
Splints/support/bandage	1
Aspiration	0
Steroid injection	0
Blood test	0
X-ray	1
Routine referral	1
Urgent referral	0
Emergency referral	0
None of these	0

Surgeon's view: An X-ray is sometimes helpful to exclude arthritis of the ankle if dorsiflexion and plantarflexion are painful. Most cases of valgus hindfoot can be corrected by orthoses, but if simple orthoses fail referral is warranted to supply more complex supports or surgery if this fails.

6

A 40-year-old man complains of pain in his Achilles tendon which comes on when running to get fit for your Well Man clinic. It is now severe and unremitting. You have examined him – the Achilles tendon region is so swollen that you cannot feel the tendon, but when laid prone with the calf squeezed the foot does plantarflex.

Simple analgesics	1
NSAIDs	1
Rest	1
Physiotherapy	1
Splints/support/bandage	1
Aspiration	0
Steroid injection	0
Blood test	0
X-ray	0
Routine referral	1
Urgent referral	0
Emergency referral	1
None of these	0

Surgeon's view: He appears to have Achilles tendonitis, which should be treated by rest, orthotics (heel raise) anti-inflammatories (NSAIDs and physiotherapy). If he does not settle completely routine referral for a plaster may help. If you are in doubt about a Thompson's test in this case with gross swelling, he should be referred as an emergency. The specialist will have access to ultrasound and MRI scans if he or she is also in doubt.

Injection of the first metatarsophalangeal joint

Indications

For arthritis.

Technique

With the patient supine palpate the joint.

Insert a 21-gauge needle either to the lateral or medial side of the extensor tendon. Aim to pass the needle into the joint. Inject slowly into the joint.

Usually use 2–3 ml of a combination of **either** 25 mg hydrocortisone acetate, **or** 10 mg triamcinalone, **or** 20 mg methylprednisolone with 1% lidocaine.

Frequency

Every 4–6 weeks. If there is no benefit after two or three injections then consider alternative treatment or referral.

Structures at risk

Injection directly onto bone or periosteum is exquisitely painful, so try and avoid it.

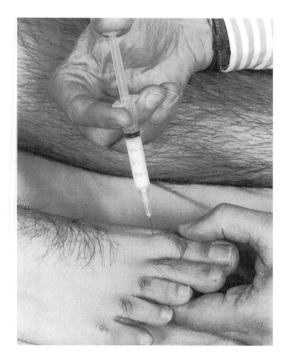

Fig. 8.11 *Injection of the first metatarsophalangeal joint*

Simple removal of toenail or nail bed ablation

Technique

Instruments needed

Tube drain, Thwaites scissors, (anvil and blade scissors), two large artery clips, forceps, McDonald dissector, scalpel and currette.

Procedure

1 Any infection should be treated with antibiotics for 5–7 days prior to surgery. Nail bed ablation should not be performed in the presence of infection, because of the risk of deep-spreading infection. In addition, local anaesthetics are often inactivated at low pH (such as occurs in infected tissues) and a few days treatment with antibiotics can usually ensure that adequate anaesthesia is obtained.

2 A ring block of local anaesthetic should be injected around the great toe. The innervation of the great toe is diffuse and the injection must be circumferential. **Under no circumstances must local anaesthetic with adrenaline be used**, as it can cause gangrene.

3 A rubber tube drain or similar is used as a tourniquet around the toe. This should be held in place with a surgical clip and should not be tied (this is to prevent accidentally leaving the tourniquet in place at the end of the procedure).

4 If phenol ablation is to be used, full precautions must be taken at this time, including the operator wearing protective clothing of gloves, glasses or visor, and protecting the skin surrounding the nail with paraffin gauze dressing.

5 The nail is removed by passing one blade of an artery forcep deep to the nail, grasping the nail and twisting it in each direction. If only a wedge of nail is to be removed then the nail should be divided longitudinally using an end-cutting beaver-type scalpel blade or a flat anvil to pass beneath the nail on to which the cutting blade closes. The use of standard sharp surgical scissors will lead to splitting of the remaining nail, and the risk of further ingrowth.

6 The surgical field is then cleaned and dried, and the paraffin gauze dressings checked. Any granulation tissue is curretted clear.

7 Small tufts of cotton wool are soaked in phenol, and placed beneath the nail fold, taking special care to treat the corner recesses of the nail where recurrent nail growth is common. In the event of accidental spillage, then rapid and thorough irrigation with saline should be applied.

8 The cotton wool applied to the nail bed should be left in place for 2 minutes. At the end of this time it is carefully removed in its entirety and the area cleansed and irrigated with a plentiful supply of saline.

9 Non-adhesive dressings are applied and a narrow crepe bandage placed around the toe before removing the clip on the tourniquet and the tourniquet itself.
10 The dressings should be soaked off after 2 days and replaced.

Notes

After simple removal of the nail, full re-growth of the nail may take up to a year.

1 Regrowth of the nail may occur after phenol ablation. This risk is increased if the phenol is not kept in a cool dark place. It should be replaced periodically as it degrades over a period of time.
2 Phenol is a very toxic fluid and must be handled and stored with great care.

9

Children ──────────────── Michael K.D. Benson

- A typical finding of bone/joint sepsis is pseudoparalysis.
- Back pain associated with scoliosis indicates serious pathology in children.
- Clicky hips rarely matter, hip instability does.
- Fifty per cent of limping children with knee pain will have hip pathology.
- Nocturnal limb pains in children are common, often transitory, and in the absence of clinical findings require reassurance.

Presenting symptoms

It is a trite but true comment that children are not just little adults. A range of conditions affects children uniquely and growth modifies the child's response to deformity, infection and injury.

Children are often better historians than their parents: when possible listen to the child's account of his or her problem and not the parent's interpretation.

Children may feel threatened by unfamiliar surroundings. While bright lights and an examination couch help the doctor, the child is almost always happier on his or her mother's lap. It is sensible always to leave the unpleasant part of an examination until the end: abduct the child's hips at the end of the examination, not at the beginning.

Children both recover and deteriorate quickly with illness. If, for example, bone or joint sepsis is suspected, it is always wise to re-examine a child a few hours later when the situation has clarified.

Orthopaedic problems in children of any age

Infection

Bone and joint infections are serious at any age and need urgent hospital admission. If the diagnosis is suspected the child should always be referred as an emergency. It is a mistake to treat blind, with antibiotics. Although it is true that a few bacteria are most commonly involved, blind antibiotic treatment may obscure the causative organism and make the correct selection of antibiotics almost impossible.

In the neonate and young infant the diagnosis of infection may be hazardous. Fever is not invariably present but the child is unhappy and listless. A typical finding is pseudoparalysis: the child does not voluntarily move the affected joint. In the case, for example, of shoulder sepsis, Erb's palsy may mistakenly be diagnosed. In a superficial joint or bone the diagnosis is usually obvious in the older child with local swelling and tenderness. In a deeply placed joint even in the older child it may be only restriction of joint movement that points to the diagnosis. Bone and joint infection is almost always blood borne and not infrequently the primary focus of infection is elusive.

Tumours

Benign bone tumours are not rare in childhood. Almost always they cause no symptoms until they present as a consequence of minor injury with a pathological fracture. Some benign tumours, like hereditary multiple exostoses, are familial.

Malignant bone and soft tissue tumours are fortunately rare in infancy and in childhood, but become slightly more common in adolescence. All bone tumours are most common about the knee where most skeletal growth takes place. Bone tumours should be suspected if pain is present both at night and day and if there is local bone thickening and tenderness. Clearly it would be inappropriate for every child with knee ache to be X-rayed, but aching unrelated to exercise or activity which causes night discomfort should trigger alarm bells.

Scoliosis

Congenital scoliosis may be apparent at birth. It is then associated with abnormalities of individual vertebrae, so that they are either partially conjoined or absent. Angular deformity may be demonstrable but rotation is often not prominent. Such vertebral anomalies may be associated with spina bifida.

It is sensible during any routine developmental check on a child to examine the spine but routine school screening for scoliosis, so-called 'schooliosis', is no longer practised. The problem is that many children have mild spinal asymmetry and spinal surgeons were overwhelmed by demand when all such children were referred to them!

If any spinal curve is detected, provided it is trivial it does not need referral. It is however essential that the child be sequentially evaluated by the general practitioner and if there is any hint of progression then clearly referral is appropriate. Particular care should be taken in adolescence when rapid curve progression may develop.

It should be noted that it is unusual for children to complain of back pain and if back pain is associated with scoliosis there is a high likelihood of a significant underlying spinal problem. The combination of pain and scoliosis demands specialist referral as spinal infection, tumour or intrathecal abnormality may underlie this combination of complaints.

Rickets and metabolic bone disease

Dietary rickets is vanishingly rare in the UK now. Familial vitamin D-resistant rickets is less rare and, unlike children with dietary rickets, those with hypophosphataemic rickets are bright and cheerful and have no proximal muscle weakness. Pronounced deformity in the weight-bearing lower limbs is common, with anterolateral femoral bowing and internal torsion with bowing of the tibia being the most common deformities. The bony deformities are symmetrical and progressive unless halted by diagnosis and appropriate treatment. Similar bone deformities may occur in children with renal impairment.

Any child of abnormal stature, whether too tall or too small or with limb/trunk length disproportion, should be referred to a growth expert, as there are a plethora of rare skeletal dysplasias with additional variants being regularly described.

Age-related problems

Infancy

Congenital anomalies

Most orthopaedic problems are visually apparent. Extra digits, syndactyly and missing parts are easily seen. A deep dimple or pit may reflect an underlying bony deficit. Deep dimples in the buttocks, for example, may suggest an absent sacrum. Deformities at the hip and spine may be more difficult to detect. The spine is most easily checked with the child held prone and flopping down on the examiner's hand. It is easy to check for scoliosis. It is easy to palpate the spine and ensure there is no spinous process absence, suggesting an underlying occult spina bifida. Skin blemishes such as patches of pigmentation or hairy tufts should alert the examiner to the possibility of an underlying spinal and neurological defect. It is wise to check for postanal pits and dimples: if these are not blind ending, neurosurgical advice should be sought. It is important to remember that, in infancy, occult spinal abnormalities may not be associated with a neurological deficit but if abnormal cord tethering is present neurological symptoms and signs may develop with growth.

It is very important to remember that if a child has one congenital anomaly there is a likelihood that there may be others.

Children are amazingly malleable after birth and postural deformity is common. The prone-lying child tends to develop hooked forefeet or metatarsus adductus. The side-lying child readily develops an eccentric skull shape, a postural scoliosis and asymmetry in hip abduction. Parents should be encouraged to alternate the sleeping position of their children.

The hips

In 1969 a circular to all doctors advised that all children's hips should be carefully examined by the manoeuvres described by Ortolani and Barlow. It was transitorily believed that this would prevent the late presentation of all children with hip dislocation. The recommendations are under review but it is currently advised that all children should have their hips examined at birth and before discharge from hospital. They should subsequently be examined at 6–8 weeks, 6–8 months and thereafter at 18–24 months. While the hip examination may be in part delegated to health visitors, it is important that all doctors who deal with children are competent in hip examination techniques. As background it is worth noting that 2% of all children have hips which are demonstrably unstable at birth. Fortunately the great majority of these resolve and need no treatment. If no screening is performed, however, one to two per 1000 are left with displaced hips and a further one to two present in later life with premature arthritis as a consequence of hip dysplasia. The fashionable term for describing the range of hip instability and dysplasia is now 'developmental dysplasia of the hip'. The important point to remember when examining the child's hip is that one is feeling to see what the relationship is between the femoral head and the acetabulum. The hip is either in joint and stable, in joint but displaceable, out of joint but reducible or out of joint and irreducible. The most common error is to feel for a click. Clicks rarely matter, instability does!

If hip instability is not recognizable at birth, within a few weeks fixed displacement of the hip joint occurs and the cardinal signs change. The child's leg may be slightly short, externally rotated and have asymmetrical thigh creases (but one in three normal children have asymmetrical thigh creases!). If the hip is displaced the critical clinical sign is restriction of abduction in flexion.

If ever there is doubt about a child's hip it is wise to refer for specialist examination. In the older child over the age of 4 months it would be entirely reasonable to refer a child for X-ray evaluation and to refer to a specialist only if the X-ray is abnormal.

It is of course worth remembering the at-risk factors for hip instability. These include oligohydramnios, an affected family member, a breech presentation and/or delivery, and foot deformity.

The knees

Knee deformities are rare at birth, but the most common would be the hyperextended or dislocated knee seen only in association with neurological abnormality or an extended breech.

The foot

By contrast foot deformities are common. The most frequent is talipes calcaneovalgus (talipes = talus + pes = ankle + foot). The calcaneovalgus foot is directed upwards and outwards and needs nothing other than simple stretching. Almost all resolve within a matter of a few weeks. As noted before, it may be associated with hip instability.

Talipes equinovarus or club foot occurs in two per 1000 children and is sometimes familial. It is increasingly recognized on antenatal ultrasound. Club feet need specialist treatment by serial stretching, strapping, plaster or physiotherapy and many will come to need surgery in the first few months of life. It is important to note that a true structural club foot will always be smaller than its counterpart and that calf wasting is an integral

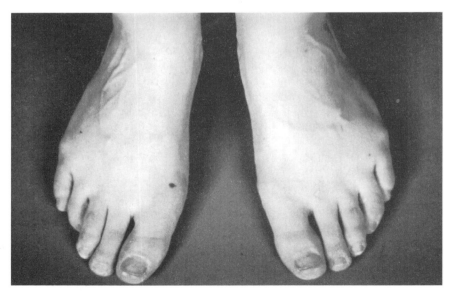

Fig. 9.1 *Curly fourth toes which very rarely require treatment*

part of the problem and cannot be augmented by simple exercise. Minor toe deformities are common: the second toe often appears high riding and needs no treatment. Curliness of the fourth and fifth toes is often familial and certainly needs no treatment in infancy.

Provided the infant's foot is supple and flexible it is unlikely to be a problem. If it is stiff and inflexible expert advice should be sought, as there may be underlying bony coalition or a neuromuscular deficit.

The toddler

Walking is a critical age of childhood development. Parents are concerned by late walking. Bottom-shuffling children frequently do not walk independently until over 18 months. Any child who has not walked by 2 years, however, needs specialist evaluation by a paediatrician to ensure there is no neuromuscular abnormality.

When children start walking many problems are highlighted. The parents are concerned by bandiness, knock-knees, intoeing, out-toeing and flat foot. It is important to remember there is a normal physiological development: most children are slightly bandy when they start to walk but they may appear to be slightly knock-kneed by the age of 2–3 years and this resolves slowly over the course of the next 4–5 years.

When assessing apparent angular deformity one should always look for symmetry. Asymmetrical knock-knee may, for example, be the consequence of partial growth arrest or injury and needs specialist referral. Provided the bones themselves appear straight and the angular deformities are slight, there is no indication for referral. In a bandy child it is sensible to measure the distance between the knees when the ankles are just touching and in the knock-knee child to measure the distance between the medial malleoli when the knees are just touching. There is rarely a cause for concern if the gap between the knees in a bandy child is 5 cm or less and in a knock-kneed child if the ankle gap is 7 cm or less.

Intoeing is common and is associated either with femoral torsion or internal tibial torsion. Both seem to be more common in lax-jointed children. Femoral torsion is simply judged by lying the child on its back with the knee flexed over the end of the couch and the hips extended. The hip can then be rotated internally and externally by rotating the leg like the hand of a clock. In general, the range of internal and external rotation is similar. Frequently it is found that the range of internal rotation considerably exceeds that of external rotation. It is this asymmetry that allows the child to sit in the TV sitting position, to walk with the toes turned in and to run with legs flicking sideways. The great majority of children need no treatment and there is spontaneous improvement over the first 7–10 years of life.

Internal tibial torsion may be judged with the child in the same position simply by dorsiflexing the foot and by checking which position the foot faces with regard to the knee. The average child will have 20 degrees of external torsion but there is a wide range of normal. It is not uncommon to see children with 40–50 degrees of internal torsion at toddler age and, surprisingly, the vast majority of these improve by school age. It is actually surprisingly uncommon for children to trip themselves up by catching one foot behind the opposite leg.

The limping child

The child who limps must always be taken seriously. The limp may reflect anything from a minor ankle sprain to hip sepsis. Beware of the child who complains of knee pain: at least 50% of such children will have a hip problem rather than a knee problem and failure to examine the hip causes considerable problems in litigation. Careful detailed analysis will usually allow the site of the problem, if not the diagnosis, to be clarified.

In the absence of trauma the hip is by far the most frequent source of the problem in the toddler. Differential diagnosis includes hip disloca-tion, sepsis, the irritable hip and Perthes' disease. The dislocated hip should readily be diagnosed by leg shortness with restricted abduction but no pain. It may be difficult to distinguish between the other three. In the presence of a healthy child it is entirely reasonable to wait a few hours and re-examine. If hip discomfort has increased, the child has become unwell and the range of hip movement has decreased, then urgent referral and admission is mandatory. Of all joints that may be affected by infection the hip is the most problematical, as infection here may lead to the destruction of the femoral head by avascular necrosis within 24 hours unless surgical decompression is urgently undertaken.

In practice, by toddler age, the signs of an infected hip are usually clear with a febrile, unwell, unhappy child and there will be little doubt that the child needs urgent admission. It is, however, difficult to distinguish between the irritable hip and Perthes' disease and certainly in the presence of a healthy child if hip movement does not improve steadily over the course of a few days referral to a specialist is appropriate on a semi-urgent basis.

The irritable hip remains one of the enigmas of childhood. It is alterna-tively known as transient synovitis and the observation hip. A small joint effusion is easily demonstrable by ultrasound and aspiration may relieve the symptoms when a tense effusion is present. Only occasionally does an irritable hip which is radiologically normal initially progress to estab-lished Perthes' disease. Idiopathic avascular necrosis or Perthes' disease, is equally enigmatic but may lead to considerable disability and needs specialist supervision.

The foot

The flat foot is physiologically normal in children under 3 years. Children need referral only if the flat footedness is associated with pain, stiffness or grossly uneven shoe wear.

The night pains of childhood

These puzzling pains may be very distressing for the child and family. Typically the 2–8-year-old child wakes at night complaining of pain in one or other limb. Mother reassures the distressed child, massages the child's leg and gives simple analgesics. Within 30 or 40 minutes the discomfort has resolved and the child sleeps to wake refreshed and bright in the morning but with a harrowed parent. The symptoms fluctuate. Pain may occur on two to three nights in succession and then be absent for two to three weeks. There is almost never significant discomfort by day and the child does not limp. Not uncommonly there is a family history. It is the variable nocturnal pattern of pain which allows the diagnosis to be made and the parents' instinctive management is almost invariably correct.

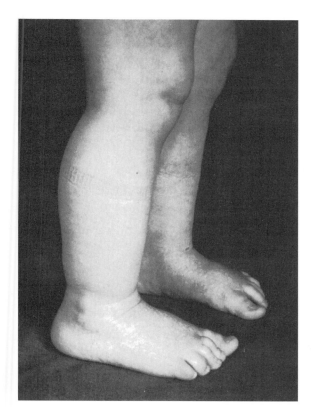

Fig. 9.2 *Infantile flat foot which rarely requires treatment*

The older child and adolescent

As the child gets older trauma becomes increasingly frequent. It is rare for an infant or young child to fracture a bone and a femoral or tibial fracture in infancy needs careful evaluation to ensure that abuse has not contributed to the injury. As the child becomes physically more adventurous fractures become more common. Boys fracture more often than girls. Stress fractures are rare before adolescence. It becomes increasingly common for children to develop discomfort where tendons insert into growing areas of bone or apophyses. Traction apophysitis at the heel (Sever's disease), at the knee (Osgood–Schlatter disease) or at the patella (Sindig–Larsen disease) are common in the 9–14-year group. Meniscal injuries become more frequent at the same age. In the child who complains of clicking or locking at the knee under the age of 10, it is not uncommon to find a pathological discoid lateral meniscus underlies the problem, but in children of adolescent age the tearing of the normal meniscus becomes increasingly more likely. It is worth remembering that pain and swelling of the knee, ankle or elbow may occur with osteochondritis dissecans: a small fragment of bone adjacent to the joint surface becomes avascular and may separate with the overlying articular carti-lage to create a loose body inside the joint.

Perthes' disease of the hip is rare after the age of 10 years. This is just as well as the prognosis deteriorates with age. Just as Perthes' disease fades in the diagnostic spectrum, so slipped upper femoral epiphysis appears. The child, often but not invariably overweight, complains of a limp and discomfort at the knee. Careful examination reveals that the leg is held in external rotation at the hip and is a little short. Movement at the hip is restricted. The usual delay between onset of symptoms and specialist referral has been shown to be 6 months. This is sad, as the slipped upper femoral epiphysis if diagnosed early can be treated simply but if diagnosed later may cause considerable management problems and lead to premature arthritis. It should be high on the list of diagnos-tic possibilities and prompt X-ray and referral organized if ever it is suspected.

Case Histories

1

You are called at six in the morning to see an 8-month-old child who is febrile and unwell. The parents complain that it hurts when his nappy is changed. The child is feverish and grizzly and screams when the cot is touched or the leg is moved.

(a) What is the presumptive diagnosis?
(b) What should be done?

Answer:
(a) Septic arthritis of the hip.
(b) Arrange urgent transfer to hospital. Give analgesics but no antibiotics.

2

A 2-year-old boy is brought in by his mother who complains that his feet are flat and he is wearing his shoes unevenly. You find him to be lax jointed and to stand with excessive heel valgus. He has supple feet and ankles. He is wearing flimsy canvas shoes.

(a) How should he be treated?
(b) Should he be referred?

Answer:
Hypermobile planovalgus feet are best treated at this age by using boots rather than flimsy shoes and specialist referral either to an orthopaedic surgeon or podiatrist is not indicated.

3

A 7-year-old child is brought by his mother to the surgery. His mother notes that he has been complaining of backache for 3 weeks. When you examine him there is a little localized mid dorsal back tenderness, a small scoliosis, moderate muscle spasm and some restricted mobility.

Should you:

(a) Reassure and review 1 week later.
(b) Arrange X-rays.
(c) Arrange routine referral.
(d) Arrange urgent referral.

Answer:
This combination of findings suggests an infective discitis and the child should be referred urgently for a specialist spinal opinion. Antibiotics should not be prescribed and it is best to allow the specialist to arrange the X-rays that are required.

4

A 5-year-old child is brought to the surgery by his mother who complains that he has been limping for 4 or 5 days. Examination reveals that the child is generally well. You find a slight limp but note that the hip has a small flexion contracture, lacks full flexion and internal rotation. The child is afebrile and otherwise well.

Should you:

(a) Refer urgently.
(b) Advise rest and re-evaluate a few hours later.
(c) Arrange X-rays.
(d) Prescribe antibiotics, anti-inflammatories or analgesics.

Answer:
The history strongly suggests an irritable hip. In a healthy child it is reasonable to advise rest at home. The child should be re-evaluated a few hours later and if the symptoms and signs acutely deteriorate then urgent referral is appropriate. If the symptoms fail to resolve the child should have a semi-urgent orthopaedic outpatient appointment to see whether the cause of the limp is simple irritability or Perthes' disease. It would be reasonable to arrange for X-rays but the presence of a normal X-ray does not exclude the possibility that avascular necrosis has occurred as radiological bone changes may not be apparent at first.

5

An 11-year-old girl is brought to the surgery by her mother complaining of unilateral knee discomfort which developed without injury and which makes her limp. On examination you find a heavy non-athletic girl with clinically normal knees.

Do you:

(a) Reassure.
(b) Arrange X-rays for her knees.
(c) Refer for specialist opinion.

Answer:
If you have not examined her hips by this stage you promptly do so remembering there is a 50% chance that her problem arises from the hip! In the presence of a normal knee a limping 11 year old has a slipped epiphysis until proved otherwise. If you confirm that hip mobility is restricted you should refer for urgent orthopaedic opinion. An antero-posterior X-ray alone may not always diagnose an epiphyseal slip and the lateral X-ray will more precisely delineate the problem.

10

Rheumatology_____ Simon Bowman

- A diagnosis of septic arthritis must be excluded in a single swollen joint.
- Loop diuretics are as potent as thiazide diuretics in inducing gout.
- Rheumatoid arthritis cannot be diagnosed until symptoms have been present for 6 weeks.
- Rheumatoid arthritis can present very similarly to polymyalgia rheumatica in older patients.
- Raynaud's phenomenon is a common presenting feature in scleroderma and systemic lupus erythematosis.

Introduction

Rheumatological problems are common in general practice. This chapter aims to provide guidelines for the initial diagnosis and management of these disorders, with a view to addressing some of the quandaries often faced by general practitioners (GPs).

The single swollen joint

Is this a septic arthritis?

- This is the first and really the only truly critical question.
- Septic arthritis demands immediate hospital referral.
- Antibiotics should not be given until after joint aspiration.

If the patient is systemically unwell, or if the joint is very painful or tender (particularly if held rigid with guarding on movement), or is red hot with overlying erythema, or lymphadenopathy is present, then an immediate hospital referral is mandatory (but see also Gout below). Aside from the dangers of septicaemia, it is now recognized that complete cartilage destruction can occur within 48 hours, and hence septic arthritis must be regarded as an orthopaedic emergency.

If this is not a septic joint then consider the following common diagnoses:

Younger person: sports injury, reactive arthritis, inflammatory arthritis.

Older person: gout, pyrophosphate arthropathy.

Is there a history of trauma?

Clearly if a fracture is suspected, an X-ray should be taken. Stress fractures through osteoporotic long bones are not uncommon in those with chronic arthritis, particularly where there is angular deformity.

1 Do not miss a scaphoid fracture; they do not always show up on an initial X-ray. If suspected refer urgently.
2 Do not miss a ruptured Achilles tendon. With the patient lying on their front, and the ankles lying free over the edge of the couch, squeeze the calf muscles. If this does not produce symmetrical plantarflexion of the ankles then this suggests the diagnosis, and an urgent orthopaedic referral should be made.
3 A history of a 'pop' during a twisting injury of the knee is character-istic of anterior cruciate ligament rupture. An effusion within 2 hours of injury indicates a probable ligament rupture.
4 Inability to fully flex the knee, or 'locking', suggests a cartilage injury.

In the acute phase appropriate treatment includes rest, NSAIDs, icepacks (or frozen peas) and a light support. A subsequent referral for physio-therapy, or to a sports injury clinic, can then be made if necessary.

If there is no history of trauma, then in **younger people** consider reactive/inflammatory arthritis, and in **older people** consider gout/pyrophosphate arthropathy.

Could this be a reactive/inflammatory arthritis?

This group of conditions can present as a single swollen joint, for example, a knee, ankle or wrist, or with several joints affected.

Is there a history of recent infection within the last few months, especially gastrointestinal or sexually transmitted disease?

Reactive arthritis

This can also present occasionally as a full-blown Reiter's syndrome (whatever the preceding infection), comprising: arthritis, conjunctivitis and urethritis.

Additional features are a rash on the penis (circinate balanitis), or palms of the hand and soles of the feet (keratoderma blennorrhagicum).

The commonest infections are:

1 Sexually transmitted disease, e.g. chlamydia.
   (a) If suspected, then assessment by a genitourinary specialist should be performed, as part of the routine procedure.
   (b) In the male, if the possibility of a sexually transmitted disease is low, a first-pass early-morning urine sent for microbiological analysis is an adequate screening test, but if pus cells are seen, a genitourinary referral is required.
   (c) A true septic arthritis due to gonococcus may also occur in patients at risk of sexually transmitted disease. Gonococcal skin pustules may be seen. If suspected (see Septic arthritis above) then urgent referral is required.
2 Gastrointestinal infections, e.g. salmonella, shigella or campylobacter.
   (a) If a gastrointestinal infection is suspected, then stool cultures should be sent and, in some localities, serological tests for salmonella and shigella may be available.
3 Occasionally other infections such as upper respiratory or urinary tract infections have been incriminated, and appropriate samples and serological investigations can be performed.

Lyme disease

This is a tick-borne infection due to *Borrelia burgdorferei* and is a rare cause of inflammatory arthritis. If there has been recent travel to a wooded area it should be suspected. Only 50% give a history of a tick-bite, but 70% have a flat, annular, red, skin rash with a sharply demarcated edge (erythema chronicum migrans) at the site of the bite. Serology can be sent and, if positive, or if strongly suspected clinically, then appropriate antibiotics should be started in consultation with the local microbiologist. If not treated early, then chronic arthritis, carditis and neurological manifestations can occur.

Inflammatory arthritis

An acute mono- or oligo-arthritis, similar to reactive arthritis, may occur in other members of the seronegative group of spondyloarthropathies.

The three to consider are:

1 **Ankylosing spondylitis**. Is there a history of back problems, or a family history of arthritis or back pain? Since uveitis is common, a history or family history of eye problems is relevant.
2 **Psoriatic arthritis**. Is there a history/family history of psoriasis. The extent of the skin disease does not correlate with the occurrence of arthritis. The scalp, elbows, natal cleft and umbilicus are common sites for subtle changes. Look for nail pitting.

3 **Inflammatory bowel disease**. Crohns disease and ulcerative colitis can both be associated with an asymmetrical mono/oligoarthritis. The severity of the arthritis is usually related to the activity of the bowel inflammation.

An ESR and/or CRP are helpful as a correlate of disease activity. A routine baseline FBC and biochemistry screen are worth doing at the same time. In general, an X-ray is unnecessary.

Use of an inflamed joint will lead to persistence of the inflammation and damage. Hence the knees and ankles should be non-weightbearing in the acute phase. Remember the importance of footwear and padding if there is inflammation of the toes. For the knee or ankle this may require non-weightbearing of the joint through bed rest, the use of crutches and, for the knee, a backslab to be worn.

If the inflammatory markers (ESR and CRP) remain raised, even after the joint has apparently settled, a return to normal activities frequently leads to a relapse.

If the degree of swelling is mild, a NSAID, an appropriate joint support and advice to rest until the swelling has resolved may be all that is required. If it fails to settle over approximately the next week, seek further advice.

If there is more marked swelling, then joint aspiration and corticosteroid injection will be required. For the larger joints, a longer acting steroid (e.g. methylprednisolone or triamcinolone) with local anaesthetic is indicated, while hydrocortisone is used for the small joints in the hands or feet.

Fluid should be sent for microscopy (including analysis for crystals) and culture. Urate crystals can often still be detected in gouty effusions sent to the hospital laboratory by overnight post.

Most patients with significant joint swelling will be referred fairly promptly following a telephone conversation between the GP and the rheumatology department. In some units, inpatient facilities for formal splintage and rest are available.

Could this be gout or pyrophosphate arthropathy?

The older person presenting with an acutely swollen big toe will not present a diagnostic challenge. However, Gout should always be suspected as a cause of any swollen joint in an older person, and can also present as a polyarticular form (10% of cases) with systemic features of fever and malaise (Figure 10.1). Atypical presentations, for example, in the acromioclavicular joints, can occur.

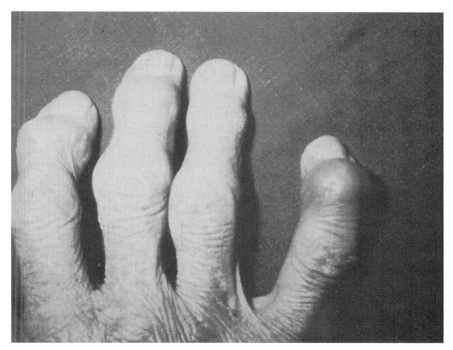

Fig. 10.1 *A gout tophus of the little finger and primary osteoarthritis*

Gout

Predisposing factors for gout

- Family history
- alcohol
- diuretics (n.b. loop diuretics are as potent as thiazides)
- smoking
- obesity
- hypertension
- ischaemic heart disease
- leukaemia
- fasting
- exercise
- trauma
- low-dose aspirin
- postoperation

Investigations

Urate crystals in synovial fluid or the presence of tophi confirms the diagnosis.

Serum urate, FBC, ESR and/or CRP (neutrophil leucocytosis and raised inflammatory markers are common, and may be extreme, e.g. ESR 100 mm/h and WCC 20 ×10^9/l, and the occasional leukaemia can present with gout). Baseline serum urea and electrolytes and creatinine should be performed, as gout can impair renal function, and the result may also influence the treatment.

Urate levels are normal in 15% of acute attacks.

Treatment of the acute attack

Rest is needed.

NSAIDs and/or colchicine are prescribed. Colchicine can either be given as high doses, e.g. 1 mg stat, and 500 μg 2–3 hourly until 10 mg is given. It may be limited by gastrointestinal intolerance (nausea or diarrhoea). It can be given more chronically at 500 μg two to three times a day. Monitoring of renal function is important in the elderly or if high doses are being given.

Local corticosteroid injection can be very effective. Occasionally the use of oral or intramuscular (or rarely intravenous) steroids may be helpful, but generally when the patient is in a hospital. Once the acute attack has settled, the urate level should be repeated.

Review the elimination of possible contributory factors, and avoid excessive consumption of foods rich in purines (red meat and wine). Beer consumption in particular is a potent contributory factor.

Treatment of chronic gout or recurrent attacks

Long-term allopurinol is indicated if:

1 There are frequent acute attacks.
2 Tophi are present.
3 Renal impairment is present secondary to gout.
4 There is a persistently high serum urate (>550 mmol/l).

This can be started at a dose of 100 mg a day and increased until the serum urate is normalized.

Allopurinol can precipitate an acute attack. Therefore, it should not be started during an acute attack, and the first 6–8 weeks after the initiation of allopurinol treatment should be covered with an anti-inflammatory drug or colchicine.

Pyrophosphate arthropathy (often called pseudogout)

Joint inflammation can also occur due to intra-articular calcium pyrophosphate deposition. Typically it occurs in the elderly on a background of osteoarthritis, and presents with a swollen knee, wrist or shoulder. Occasionally a polyarticular presentation occurs.

Investigations

The presence of chondrocalcinosis on X-ray supports the diagnosis. Calcification of the triangular cartilage of the wrist is pathognomonic, while in the knee it is less specific.

A positive result from joint aspiration is diagnostic, but the crystals are more fragile than urate crystals and can be difficult to detect. Hence a negative result does not always exclude the diagnosis.

Pseudogout is often labelled as 'an acute exacerbation of osteoarthritis'. Since the treatment is the same this may not be a critical issue. However it may mimic septic arthritis which may need to be excluded.

Serum biochemistry including calcium and phosphate, liver function tests, thyroid function and urate should be checked, as **hyperparathyroidism, hypothyroidism, gout** and **haemochromatosis** can all be associated with pseudogout.

Treatment

Rest, NSAIDs and corticosteroid injection are the basis of treatment. Unlike gout, there is no prophylactic treatment.

Polyarthritis

A specialist review at an early stage is advisable for all patients with inflammatory polyarthritis. The team of physiotherapists, occupational therapists and doctors, as well as access to support networks, are major advantages that accrue from this.

Rheumatoid arthritis (RA)

This is the commonest inflammatory arthritis. Diagnosis is based on clinical pattern recognition.

Early-morning stiffness is the hallmark of inflammatory arthritis, and may be the only feature early in the disease.

Synovitis, i.e. visibly swollen, boggy swelling of the joints, is necessary to make a diagnosis of arthritis.

Symmetrical involvement of the metacarpal (MCP) and proximal interphalangeal (PIP) joints, wrists and tendon sheaths of the hand are common (Figure 10.2). Ask about and examine the feet, as a similar process occurs and can be diagnostically helpful. Metatarsalgia and stiffness of the toes are common.

The differential diagnosis depends partly on the presentation. In general RA develops over weeks to months.

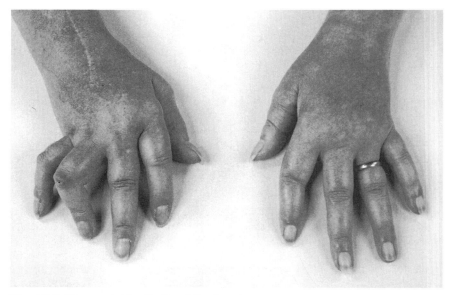

Fig. 10.2 *Rheumatoid arthritis of the hands*

It can present at any age, but with peaks after childbirth and the menopause in women, and during the winter months. Since osteoarthritis is common, its presence (e.g. bony swelling of the PIP and distal interphalangeal (DIP) joints) does not exclude the diagnosis.

Connective tissue disorders can rarely mimic RA. Think of these if features of **Raynaud's phenomenon, systemic lupus erythematosus (SLE)** or **scleroderma** are present (see below), and if suspected check for anti-nuclear antibody (ANA). Other rare conditions are primary biliary cirrhosis, chronic active hepatitis and haemochromatosis. Many psoriatic arthritis patients can have similar features to seronegative RA.

Bilateral carpal tunnel syndrome is an important presentation of polyarthritis, for example, RA/scleroderma (see below). If present check thyroid function, and dipstick the urine to exclude diabetes.

Acute presentation

Acute viral arthritis can present identically to RA, but in general this is self-limiting over a few weeks. The two viruses to test for are parvovirus B19 and rubella.

RA cannot be diagnosed until symptoms have been present for 6 weeks.

Polymyalgic presentation

RA can present very similarly to polymyalgia rheumatica, particularly in older patients. It may not be possible to differentiate the two until more typical synovitis occurs.

Investigations

Many patients believe that the presence of rheumatoid factor equates with the diagnosis of RA. It can, however, be found in other inflammatory arthritides and with some infections, and at low titres in about 5% of healthy individuals. A negative rheumatoid factor does not exclude the diagnosis.

FBC: a normochromic, normocytic anaemia and increased platelets are common in active RA.

ESR and/or CRP are commonly raised. Occasionally they can be normal or only slightly raised, despite active synovitis.

Biochemistry and urinalysis: a raised alkaline phosphatase and gGT are common. If there is significant proteinuria or haematuria, this may suggest a rare vasculitic condition.

X-rays of the hands and feet are usually normal in early disease. Erosions, if they are going to occur, are nearly always evident within the first 2 years of disease. X-rays are worth doing at presentation and at 1 year, but may be worth leaving until the specialist review.

Treatment

The finding that erosions and joint damage occur early has changed rheumatological practice. Disease-modifying anti-rheumatic drugs (DMARDs) are now used early in treating RA to try and control acute inflammation, and with the secondary aim of slowing the rate of progression of disease. It must be said, however, that it is unclear at present precisely how effective these agents are in influencing the long-term outcome. In general these are started with specialist advice, but hydroxychloroquine 200 mg b.d. (with an ophthalmological assessment required initially and at yearly intervals) or sulphasalazine (ask about sulphonamide allergies, start at 500 mg o.d. and increase to 1 g b.d. over 4–8 weeks, with FBC and LFT after 2 weeks, at monthly intervals for 6 months, and 3 monthly thereafter) are occasionally started in the community. It takes 3 months to assess whether they are effective.

There is rarely such a thing as a short course of steroids in RA (unlike asthma). Steroids usually require reduction at 1 mg/month in inflammatory arthritis (i.e. from 10 mg down to 0 mg takes 10 months). Hence do not start oral steroids unless you are prepared to continue them indefinitely. A better alternative if you are desperate is IM Depo-medrone 120 mg.

Dry eyes or mouth in RA is usually due to inflammation in the salivary glands (secondary Sjögren's syndrome). Artificial tears are effective treatment for the eyes, but a dry mouth is more difficult to treat. Lozenges and sprays are available (see the British National Formulary).

Polymyalgia rheumatica (PMR) and giant cell arteritis (GCA)

These conditions are rare under age 50.

The classical case of PMR is of pain and stiffness across the shoulder blades and pelvic girdle, which is worse in the mornings, and with a high ESR.

The response to steroids (prednisolone 15 mg o.d. initially in PMR) is often dramatic.

Synovitis can occasionally occur.

If there is headache, visual disturbance, jaw claudication, tenderness of the temporal arteries or systemic symptoms, then **giant cell (temporal) arteritis** may be present, with a risk of sudden blindness. In this case the dose of prednisolone is 45–60 mg/day. In general, emergency advice from a specialist will be sought in these circumstances. Temporal artery biopsy may be indicated.

Unfortunately many patients do not fit this neat pattern, but have borderline symptoms and ESRs. It can be extremely difficult to be certain of the diagnosis in these circumstances. If in doubt, a telephone discussion with a rheumatologist prior to starting corticosteroids should be obtained (but may not make it any easier).

Polymyositis (check creatinine phosphokinase), **myeloma** (check immunoglobulin electrophoresis and urinary Bence Jones protein) and **hypothyroidism/hyperthyroidism** should be excluded.

Regimes for steroid reduction vary, but with PMR, after 4–8 weeks as symptoms resolve and the ESR falls, the dose can be decreased to 12.5 mg and then 10 mg at monthly intervals. Below 10 mg the dose can be reduced at 1-mg steps. Remember, most patients with PMR are on steroids for about 18 months to 2 years, sometimes longer (5 years or more with giant cell arteritis), and with a significant recurrence rate. i.e. **slowly does it**. If symptoms recur and the ESR goes up, increase to the previous satisfactory dose for a few months before reducing the dose again.

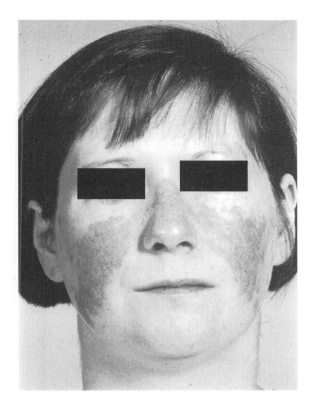

Fig. 10.3 *'Butterfly' rash in systemic lupus erythematosis*

Connective tissue disorders

Raynaud's phenomenon is a common presenting feature in two conditions: scleroderma and systemic lupus erythematosus (SLE). Both are relatively **rare** and much commoner in women than men. SLE is about 10 times less common than RA, but tends to occur in a younger age group (Figure 10.3).

The patient must be referred.

Overlap syndromes (e.g. mixed connective tissue disease, associated with anti-RNP antibodies) have been described.

Scleroderma

This is characterized by waxy thickening of the skin (especially hands and face) and internal organs. The typical age group is 30–50 years. A non-erosive synovitis can occur that is slightly atypical for RA. The patient may be unable to make a fist or open the mouth wide.

CREST syndrome is one variant with a more benign prognosis:

- Calcinosis
- Raynauds
- Esophageal dysmotility (food gets stuck)
- Sclerodactyly
- Telangiectasia (particularly facial).

Anticentromere antibodies (ACA) are often present.

Systemic sclerosis refers to a more severe variant with significant internal organ involvement. Scl-70 antibodies may be present.

- Gastrointestinal (GI) dysmotility can occur throughout the GI tract.
- Lung fibrosis is common (check a chest X-ray and lung function tests).
- Renal disease is a common cause of death (check blood pressure and renal function, including urinalysis, regularly).
- Cardiac involvement (e.g. pericarditis) can also occur.
- Sudden hypertensive crisis can occur (responds to ACE- inhibition). Steroid treatment or its withdrawal can trigger this.
- Pulmonary hypertension is a serious and potentially fatal complication.

Investigations

Check FBC, ESR, RhF, ANA, ENA (antibodies to extractable nuclear antigens: RNP is often positive), routine biochemistry and urinalysis. Specialist investigations include anticentromere antibodies (ACA) and Scl-70 antibodies.

Treatment

Keep warm, especially the hands and feet.

Nifedipine SR 10 mg b.d. is prescribed initially (but patients can be very sensitive to dose titration, both up and down). Diltiazem is an alternative. In severe cases (e.g. with digital ulceration or gangrene) sympathectomy/IV prostacyclin can be useful when treating in hospital.

SLE

This condition typically occurs in a young female.

Acute SLE, especially if there is systemic, renal, haematological or vasculitic abnormalities, requires immediate specialist advice and emergency referral. Close collaboration between the GP and specialist is required.

This condition can suddenly flare up, even after years of relative inactivity.

Features

- General malaise.
- Butterfly rash, photosensitivity, alopecia.

- Arthritis/arthralgia (they may complain of severe joint pain without obvious synovitis – think of SLE in this situation!).
- Raynaud's phenomenon.
- Pyrexia of unknown origin.
- Pleurisy/pericarditis.
- mouth ulcers.
- Epilepsy, depression/psychosis.

Investigations

- FBC (lymphopenia, neutropenia, thrombocytopenia, haemolytic anaemia).
- ESR (high in active disease).
- CRP (normal unless there is infection or serositis).
- Biochemistry (to check for renal and liver function derangements).
- Urinalysis (haematuria/proteinuria with renal involvement. If casts/proteinuria/haematuria are present, check a 24-hour urine for protein, and creatinine clearance – which needs a paired blood sample.) Proteinuria over 0.5 g/day is very significant.
- MSU (? casts).

These results will be available on the same or following day. Immunological investigations that should be put in train are:

- ANA. This is common in SLE but not specific. Low titres are frequent in the healthy elderly and in RA patients. Conversely, an ANA should be done in seronegative RA.
- Anti-double stranded DNA antibodies/DNA binding (raised in active SLE).
- Complement C3 and C4 (may be low).
- ENA (antibodies to extractable nuclear antigens; anti-Ro, anti-La and/or anti-Sm may be positive even with a negative ANA).

The Antiphospholipid syndrome is recognized as associated with SLE, and leads to **thrombotic events, recurrent abortions,** and **thrombocytopenia**. Check for the presence of both: antiphospholipid antibodies (anticardiolipin antibodies) and lupus anticoagulant (send clotting screen).

Treatment (in brief)

Treatment for skin/arthritis includes NSAIDs, topical corticosteroid cream, complete sun block, and consider hydroxychloroquine 200 mg o.d./b.d. Azathioprine can be helpful in conjunction with specialist advice.

Vasculitis/renal disease/cytopenia, if present, requires immediate referral, and specialist treatment includes corticosteroids (which may be high dose oral/IV), and/or oral/pulsed IV cyclophosphamide. Some controversy exists over when/if to switch to azathioprine, for example, after

6–12 months if the clinical condition remains stable.

Lower dose corticosteroids are used for persistent malaise, fever, pleurisy, pericarditis or haemolytic anaemia. In general start with a higher dose and reduce, again in conjunction with specialist advice.

Prophylactic aspirin is given if cardiolipin antibody is persistently raised or lupus anticoagulant is present. Consider warfarin if there are serious or recurrent thrombotic events.

Sulphonamides and penicillins may precipitate flares.

Swollen joints in children

An acute arthritis in children can occur following viral infections, particularly parvovirus, rubella, mumps and chickenpox (occasionally post vaccination). In reality a significantly swollen joint in a child will lead to emergency referral.

For acute monoarthritis see the adult protocol above, but also check a viral screen, throat swab and antistreptolysin titre, urinalysis, rheumatoid factor and an ANA.

Henoch–Schönlein purpura is a rare cause of arthritis, nephritis, vasculitic rash and abdominal pain, particularly in children. Some have a raised level of IgA in the blood.

Pauciarticular (i.e. four or less joints involved) juvenile chronic arthritis can be associated with **asymptomatic** iridocyclitis that can lead to **blindness** if not picked up. The highest rate is in females with arthritis developing in early childhood (<5 years) with ANA +ve disease.

Low back pain

Most low back pain is mechanical and is managed with rest, analgesics, NSAIDs and physiotherapy/osteopathy.

Unremitting pain (think of malignancy), early-morning stiffness, sphincter disturbance and systemic malaise are all triggering features for further investigation and referral. If FBC/ESR/biochemistry (especially alkaline phosphatase) are abnormal, **even in a well person**, this should also trigger warning signals, and so these are worth checking before referral.

Spondyloarthropathy (e.g. ankylosing spondylitis)

An initial specialist opinion is desirable, and also worthwhile in order to gain access to the specialist team.

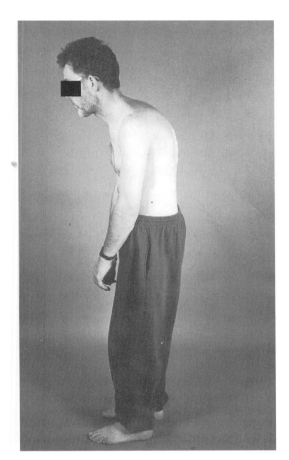

Fig. 10.4 *The typical appearance of ankylosing spondylitis*

Features

- There may be a family history.
- Early-morning stiffness.
- Waking at 02.00–04.00 h with pain.
- Chest pain due to thoracic spinal involvement.
- Onset may occur gradually in teens/young adulthood.
- Worsens with rest.
- Uveitis is common (30%).
- Plantar fasciitis/Achilles tendonitis and peripheral joint disease can all be presenting features.

Ask about a history/family history of psoriatic arthritis, inflammatory bowel disease or reactive arthritis, as these can cause a spondyloarthropathy identical to ankylosing spondylitis. On examination pain is worse on extension of the spine, while lateral flexion may be the first affected movement.

Investigations

FBC/ESR/CRP/biochemistry (the ESR and CRP are often normal, especially if there is predominantly spinal disease).

Consider an X-ray of the pelvis for sacroiliitis, preferably at the hospital where a referral would be likely to occur.

Consider checking for HLA-B27. It is found in 95% of cases of ankylosing spondylitis and 40–70% of psoriatic/reactive arthritis patients, but also in **10%** of the general population. It is not worth doing if there is radiological evidence of spondylitis, and is more useful to help exclude the diagnosis rather than to prove it.

Treatment

NSAIDs will give a marked improvement after 1–2 weeks if the diagnosis is relevant.

Physiotherapy, hydrotherapy and exercises are all prescribed.

Sulphasalazine, azathioprine or methotrexate can be considered if peripheral joint involvement is present. Oral steroids are usually ineffective in inflammatory spondylitis.

Antimalarials are contraindicated in psoriatic arthritis, as they can worsen the skin disease.

Conclusions

Close communication between the general practitioner and the rheumatologist is an important part of the management of these disorders, both with regard to the acute presentation, and the ongoing management of these generally chronic conditions.

The involvement of the rheumatology team, including nurses, physiotherapists and occupational therapists, is a critical resource that should not be underestimated, as is access to the support groups which exist for many of these conditions.

Case Histories

1

A 59-year-old man with rheumatoid arthritis presented, complaining of severe pain in his right elbow associated with substantial redness and swelling. There was no history of trauma and he felt well in himself.

Simple analgesics	1
NSAIDs	0

Rest	1
Physiotherapy	1
Splints/support/bandages	1
Aspiration	1
Steroid injection	0
Blood test	1
X-ray	1
Routine referral	0
Urgent referral	0
Emergency referral	1
None of these	0

Answers: His GP treated him initially with analgesics and a combination of amoxycillin and clavulanic acid, and subsequently with a cephalosporin. There was no improvement and he was referred to hospital as an emergency following a telephone conversation with the on-call registrar. Aspiration of the joint yielded frank pus from which *Staphylococcus aureus* was grown. The elbow improved during 2 weeks of intravenous flucloxacillin treatment. Following this a further 4 weeks of oral therapy was given, along with physiotherapy to get the elbow moving again.

2

A 30-year-old man developed an acutely swollen left knee. He had previously had uveitis and was HLA-B27+ve. He denied any recent infection or risk of sexually transmitted disease. On examination the knee was warm and distended but not red, and he could incompletely flex and extend it with some discomfort.

Simple analgesics	1
NSAIDs	1
Rest	1
Physiotherapy	1
Splints/support/bandages	1
Aspiration	1
Steroid injection	1
Blood test	1
X-ray	0
Routine referral	0
Urgent referral	1
Emergency referral	1
None of these	0

Answers: In view of his previous history and HLA status, a B27 arthropathy of some kind was clearly the likeliest diagnosis. An FBC,

ESR, CRP and baseline biochemistry were taken in the surgery. Urinalysis showed blood and protein and so an MSU was sent. He was started on an NSAID and given some crutches, and an appointment to see the local rheumatologist the following morning was made. At that time the joint was aspirated and injected with Depo-medrone. The ESR was 100 mm/h, and the CRP 250 units (normal less than 6), while there was no growth from the MSU. The patient was admitted and the knee splinted for 1 week. After this and subsequent physiotherapy, he settled completely with the ESR returning to normal. Pelvic X-ray showed sacroiliitis. An EMU showed pus cells, so that despite the history he was given a course of a tetracycline by the genitourinary specialist.

3

A 65-year-old nun returned from a trip to a convent in the Italian countryside. She subsequently developed a swollen right knee.

Simple analgesics	1
NSAIDs	1
Rest	1
Physiotherapy	0
Splints/support/bandages	1
Aspiration	1
Steroid injection	0
Blood test	1
X-ray	1
Routine referral	0
Urgent referral	0
Emergency referral	0
None of these	0

Answers: Aspiration of the joint showed only a few pus cells. As pseudogout was suspected an X-ray was performed, and osteoarthritis but not chondrocalcinosis was seen. FBC, biochemistry, urate and thyroid function tests were normal. Following rest and an NSAID her knee had improved. The area she had visited in Italy was in wooded countryside, and sleeping conditions at the convent were basic. She was uncertain whether she might have been bitten by a tick but thought it quite likely. She had not had a skin rash. Just to be on the safe side, the GP also sent paired blood samples for Lyme serology, and was telephoned by the local microbiologist to be told it was strongly positive. Treatment with antibiotics was instituted and she had no further problems.

4

A 70-year-old man with severe ischaemic heart disease, who is taking 10 different drugs including two forms of diuretics, developed a red, hot, swollen, painful big toe.

Simple analgesics	0
NSAIDs	1
Rest	0
Physiotherapy	0
Splints/support/bandages	0
Aspiration	1
Steroid injection	1
Blood test	1
X-ray	0
Routine referral	0
Urgent referral	0
Emergency referral	0
None of these	0

Answers: A clinical diagnosis of gout was made. Serum urate was 50% above the upper limit of the normal range. The serum creatinine was also raised, and an FBC showed a neutrophilia with a high ESR. He was started on b.d. colchicine, but could not tolerate it, and so an NSAID was prescribed. The GP injected adjacent to his big toe with a small amount of hydrocortisone and lignocaine. The creatinine and urate were carefully monitored and after 10 days his symptoms had settled. The NSAID was continued, and after 3 more weeks allopurinol was started and increased at monthly intervals until his urate was within the normal range. He has had no further acute attacks.

5

A 79-year-old lady came to her GP complaining of an acute onset of severe pain and swelling of the left wrist. Otherwise she felt well in herself. On examination, as well as the swollen wrist, osteoarthritic changes in the hand were noted.

Simple analgesics	1
NSAIDs	1
Rest	1
Physiotherapy	0
Splints/support/bandages	1
Aspiration	1
Steroid injection	1
Blood test	1

X-ray	1
Routine referral	0
Urgent referral	1
Emergency referral	0
None of these	0

Answers: The GP was concerned about a septic arthritis, but after discussion with the on-call registrar about the possibility of pyrophosphate arthropathy agreed to wait until the following day. In the meantime a FBC, ESR, biochemistry, urate and thyroid function were sent. A small amount of fluid was successfully aspirated from the swelling over the wrist and sent for analysis. The patient was given a wrist support, and an NSAID and analgesia were prescribed. She was sent for an X-ray to the hospital. The following day she had improved slightly. The aspirate showed pus cells, but no organisms, and no crystals were seen. The ESR was slightly raised but the other blood tests unremarkable. X-ray showed chondrocalcinosis. It was decided that referral was now unnecessary as the diagnosis of pseudogout seemed likely, and the patient was improving.

6

A 33-year-old woman with a 3-month-old baby presented with a 4-week history of pain and swelling of her hands, shoulders and knees, associated with profound early morning stiffness.

Simple analgesics	1
NSAIDs	1
Rest	1
Physiotherapy	0
Splints/support/bandages	1
Aspiration	0
Steroid injection	0
Blood test	1
X-ray	0
Routine referral	0
Urgent referral	1
Emergency referral	0
None of these	0

Answers: In view of the relatively acute history of what was probably rheumatoid arthritis in a young woman with a new baby, an urgent appointment was made, and she was seen 3 days later. The GP had sent off an FBC, ESR, CRP, biochemistry, rheumatoid factor, ANA and a viral screen. Urinalysis was negative. When she was seen she had active inflammation of her joints. The ESR was 100 mm/h, CRP 250 units and the ALK was raised. X-rays of the hands and feet were normal. She declined hospital admission in view of her young baby, and was treated with an intravenous infusion of 1 g methylprednisolone, and started on sulphasalazine. The rheumatoid factor subsequently came back with a titre of 1 in 2560, and the viral screen (which included parvovirus and rubella) was negative. She responded extremely well to sulphasalazine treatment.

7

A 53-year-old lady presented with a 6-week history of mild aching in the shoulder blades and thighs, particularly in the morning. She was also aware of some swelling of the sternoclavicular joints, low back pain, and MCP joints. An ESR was 45 mm/h.

Simple analgesics	0
NSAIDs	1
Rest	0
Physiotherapy	0
Splints/support/bandages	0
Aspiration	0
Steroid injection	0
Blood test	1
X-ray	1
Routine referral	0
Urgent referral	0
Emergency referral	0
None of these	0

Answers: The GP was concerned about the possibility of polymyalgia rheumatica (PMR), but since both the symptoms and ESR were borderline, decided to start an NSAID and seek an urgent outpatient review. Thyroid function tests, a creatinine kinase, rheumatoid factor, ANA, immunoglobulin electrophoresis and urinary Bence Jones protein were all negative. When seen by the specialist, the possibility of a seronegative spondyloarthropathy was also raised, but there was no sacroiliitis on X-ray, and she was HLA-B27 negative. She had no symptoms or signs to suggest giant cell arteritis, and it was felt that a temporal artery biopsy, although not unreasonable, would be unlikely to be positive. After some deliberation, she was started on 15 mg prednisolone EC, and after 48 hours reported a dramatic improvement. A presumptive diagnosis of PMR was made.

8

A 38-year-old lady presented with a 2-month history of worsening features of bilateral carpal tunnel syndrome, Raynaud's phenomenon, and stiffness of the joints in the hands with inability to make a fist.

Simple analgesics	0
NSAIDs	1
Rest	0
Physiotherapy	0
Splints/support/bandages	1
Aspiration	0
Steroid injection	1
Blood test	0
X-ray	0
Routine referral	0
Urgent referral	1
Emergency referral	0
None of these	0

Answers: In view of the relatively acute onset of carpal tunnel syndrome and Raynaud's phenomenon, the GP was concerned about a connective tissue disorder, and arranged an urgent rheumatology appointment. Otherwise the patient felt well, and the remainder of the examination was unremarkable, including her blood pressure. A FBC, biochemistry, urinalysis and thyroid function tests were all normal. The ESR was raised at 55. The GP injected her carpal tunnels and prescribed futura wrist supports to be worn at night, and an NSAID. Subsequently a rheumatoid factor came back as negative, and the ANA borderline positive at 1 in 160. ENA showed a positive anti-RNP antibody. When seen by the rheumatologist, she was unable to make a fist, and the skin on her hands appeared tight (sclerodactyly), with moderate synovitis. Examination of her chest, heart, abdomen and blood pressure was still unremarkable, although she had evidence of dry eyes and mouth. A chest X-ray, lung function tests and an echocardiogram were all normal. Anticentromere antibodies were negative, but Scl-70 was positive. A diagnosis of mixed connective tissue disease was made, comprising synovitis, Raynaud's phenomenon, carpal tunnel syndrome, sclerodactyly and a positive anti-RNP antibody. She was advised to keep her hands warm, and started on nifedipine SR 10 mg b.d. for the Raynaud's phenomenon, and D-penicillamine for the synovitis (as there is some evidence that it also slows the progression of sclerosis in these conditions). Regular review has been arranged to monitor her progress, and in particular whether she develops into systemic sclerosis. An urgent bilateral carpal tunnel decompression has been performed, as the injections were only of short-term benefit.

9

A 22-year-old woman presented complaining of general malaise following a trip to Majorca. On examination she was unwell, pyrexial and had a butterfly rash, and urinalysis showed protein 4+ and blood 3+.

Simple analgesics	0
NSAIDs	0
Rest	0
Physiotherapy	0
Splints/support/bandages	0
Aspiration	0
Steroid injection	0
Blood test	0
X-ray	0
Routine referral	0
Urgent referral	0
Emergency referral	1
None of these	0

Answers: The GP phoned the on-call rheumatologist who reviewed her that day, and admitted her immediately. Investigations showed a high ESR, and moderate thrombocytopenia, neutropenia and lymphopenia, with a raised serum creatinine, but only a mildly raised CRP. A septic screen was sent, and a 24-hour urine collection for protein and creatinine was started. An MSU showed an active sediment. A diagnosis of acute SLE was made, but with the possibility of superadded infection, and she was given 60 mg of prednisolone EC, and started on an intravenous cephalosporin. The following day a bone marrow aspiration was performed which showed an active marrow, and the preliminary septic screen result proved negative. She was treated with pulsed intravenous methylprednisolone, and subsequently IV cyclophosphamide pulses. Her renal function and blood indices returned to normal, and it was decided to hold off renal biopsy.

10

A 3-year-old boy was brought to his GP by his mother who had noticed a limp. On examination his left knee was swollen.

Simple analgesics	0
NSAID's	1
Rest	1
Physiotherapy	1
Splints/support/bandages	1
Aspiration	1
Steroid injection	1
Blood test	1
X-ray	0
Routine referral	0
Urgent referral	0
Emergency referral	1
None of these	0

Answers: The boy's GP referred him immediately to hospital, where admission, joint aspiration and corticosteroid injection, splintage, NSAID syrup, and subsequent physiotherapy and hydrotherapy led to complete resolution of his symptoms. The ESR, which had been raised, returned to the normal range. Unfortunately no ANA was performed, and no ophthalmology assessment was arranged. Six months later the boy presented again with problems with his vision, and after ophthalmology referral was found to have a chronic iridocyclitis with cataract formation. An ANA was strongly positive.

The author would like to thank his colleagues Dr Paul Wordsworth and Dr Alastair Mowat for their helpful advice and suggestions during the preparation of this chapter.

11

Exercises and postoperative recommendations ———— Jane Moser

Introduction

Exercise in the treatment of musculoskeletal disorders is undervalued and underused. Patients are increasingly discontented with tablets as a panacea and are seeking alternatives. Giving positive, specific advice and exercise does not only have a physical effect but also a psychological one. Patients feel involved and can develop a sense of control and responsibility for their problem. What do you advise when you are confronted by a patient in a busy surgery? Do you feel that you have any positive advice for a patient with low back pain for example, or do you feel there is nothing you (or they) can do? Your attitude and behaviour (along with anyone that they may come in contact with) will influence how a person will perceive and react to their musculoskeletal disorder. But you, as their doctor, definitely have an influence ('the Doctor said. . . . .') which may be almost impossible to alter!

This chapter aims to give an overview of simple advice and exercises that can be shown to patients with orthopaedic problems. They are presented by regional areas of the body, as ordered in the previous text (i.e. shoulder, elbow, wrist, cervical spine, lumbar spine, hip, knee, foot and ankle). Each area also has a section on general postoperative guidelines for common orthopaedic operations.

The exercises have been divided into programmes depending on the patient's predominant presentation. This approach is simplistic and limited to relatively straightforward orthopaedic problems. There is no one, universal, effective exercise for each area of the body. Exercises are selected as a result of assessment findings and the format used here attempts to guide you to appropriate exercises. Not all the exercises in a selected programme may be necessary and it is envisaged that there will not be the time to show more than two or three exercises. However, it is difficult to shorten the exercise programmes further, without ignoring key movements or muscles that commonly need re-education in orthopaedics. Therefore, following your examination, choose the movement which appears the most frequently restricted in terms of stiffness or weakness. Ideally only a few exercises (three to five maximum) should be given and realistic goals set. This, combined with written information, will improve compliance. These programmes have been written for you, not for the patient. They can be viewed as a library and the information used to create patient information and exercise sheets if you wish.

The exercises can be regarded as 'first aid'. They have been selected because they:

- are relatively simple to teach and perform;
- involve little or no equipment;
- can be shown easily in a primary care setting.

Discrimination between sensations of unaccustomed exercise and the patient's presenting symptoms must be made. Sensations of stiffness, aching, stretching, tightness, tiredness can be regarded as normal, particularly if the patient has not had any recent activity or has had the problem for a long time. However, as a general rule **pain should not progressively worsen** during or after these exercises, and this warning must be given. If pain/symptoms are worsening with the selected exercises:

- check the exercise is being performed correctly;
- reduce the number of repetitions and/or;
- change the exercise (e.g. weightbearing to non-weightbearing);
- stop the exercises and reassess analgesia and management.

Although the exercises appear simple, sometimes patients need encouragement and help to do them and to do them correctly. Refer patients to a chartered physiotherapist if they:

- are not making progress with simple exercises;
- require comprehensive rehabilitation;
- have severe and/or complicated presentations.

Physiotherapy assessment involves a detailed analysis of the neuromuscular skeletal system and commonly lasts for 40 minutes. Attention will also be given to the patient's lifestyle, psychological status and motivation. Exercise is a core treatment modality, but additional treatment techniques can also be given, such as:

- manual therapy (mobilizations, manipulation, soft tissue techniques);
- strapping and/or splintage;
- electrotherapy;
- education and advice.

Normally 20–30 minute physiotherapy appointments will be given for follow-up appointments which comprise feedback, reassessment and treatment. Therefore these simple exercises are no substitute for assessment and treatment by a chartered physiotherapist.

In addition to advice and exercises, each area of the body has a section an postoperative management of patients following common orthopaedic surgery. This is a general overview and will depend on:

- the type of surgical technique;
- the patient's general health and functional demands;
- the surgeon's beliefs/attitude to rehabilitation;
- the resources available.

As a result of these factors, large differences in the postoperative management of patients may be found. These guidelines can only be general in nature and primarily represent local practice (Oxford), especially as there appears to be little literature concerning the effects of postoperative regimes (protocols). Specific queries regarding postoperative management of patients must be directed to the surgical unit.

Shoulder

General advice for people with shoulder problems

If pain is experienced at night suggest:

- pillow/rolled towel under arm at night if lying on back or
- pillows in front (like a bolster) if lying on pain-free side.

Shoulder exercises

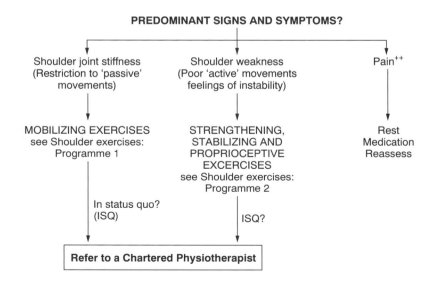

Shoulder mobilizing exercises

Shoulder Programme 1

Signs and symptoms are predominantly joint stiffness.

Advice: It may be helpful to do these exercises after the application of local heat (e.g. warm bath, shower, hot water bottle; see Appendix 11.1).

Pendulum
Leaning forwards (with support if necessary)
Let arm hang down, relaxed
Swing arm
(i)   forward and back
(ii)   side to side
(iii) around in circles (both ways)
Repeat 5–10 times each movement

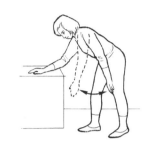

Scapula movements
Sitting, keep arms relaxed
Bring shoulders up and forwards
Then roll them 'down' and backwards
Repeat 5–10 times

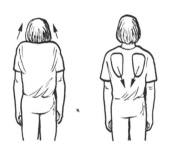

Assisted elevation in lying
Lying on back
Support arm with other hand at wrist
Lift arms overhead
Can start with elbows bent
Repeat 5–10 times

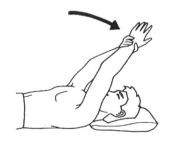

Lateral rotation
Sitting holding a stick (rolling pin, umbrella)
Keep affected side elbow into body throughout
Push with unaffected side, so hand of affected side is moving away from midline
Repeat 5–10 times
(Can be done lying down)

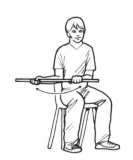

Hand behind back

Place hand behind body
Gently assist it with unaffected hand
Or use a towel/belt to pull it up back
Repeat 5–10 times

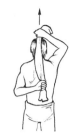

NB: This is often the last movement to return
– do not force if painful (rather than stiff)

Shoulder strengthening and stabilizing exercises

Shoulder Programme 2

Signs and symptoms are predominantly of weakness. Test and compare to the other side. What is weak?

Advice: Patients should not experience pain but may feel muscle discomfort.

Lateral rotators – glenohumeral

Sit or stand
Elbow bent and close to body
Use other hand (or wall/doorway) to stop
movement
Attempt to push affected wrist away from
body
Keep elbow in
Do not let movement occur
Hold for 10 seconds
Repeat 10–30 times
Progress this to using an elastic cord
Allow the hand to move outwards (keep
elbow close still)
Control the movement out *and back in*
Repeat 30 times

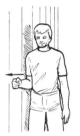

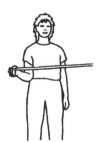

Medial rotators – glenohumeral

Sit or stand
Elbow bent and close to body
Use other hand (or wall/doorway) to stop
movement
Attempt to pull wrist towards stomach
Do not let movement occur
Hold for 10 seconds
Repeat 10–30 times

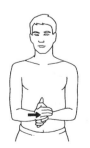

Progress this to using an elastic cord
Allow the hand to move inwards (keep
elbow close still)
Control the movement out *and back in*
Repeat 30 times

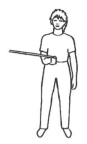

Scapula stabilization
In sitting, standing, any position
Roll shoulder blade down and back gently
Keep it there
Hold for 10 seconds
Repeat 10–30 times
Try and do this regularly through the day

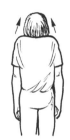
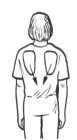

Weightbearing strengthening/ proprioception
On all fours
Take weight forwards through arms
Then try and lift UNaffected arm
Stretch *unaffected* arm in different
directions
Keep balance on other arm
Repeat 10 times

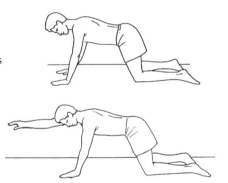

Postoperative management and advice

Shoulder replacement

These patients will be in hospital for approximately 10 days and will
start rehabilitation with the physiotherapist and occupational therapist
within 2–3 days. Outpatient physiotherapy is normally arranged for
discharge and the patient will have a home-exercise programme.

Certain movements may be restricted for up to 3 months if soft tissue
reconstruction (e.g. rotator cuff repair or lengthening) has also been
performed. The patient with a standard hemiarthroplasty or total shoulder
replacement can wean themselves out of the sling and attempt activities at
waist level as they feel able. However, early movement should be encouraged. The patient's ability to move the arm against gravity in the long term

depends on whether the rotator cuff is functional (it is often damaged and irreparable) and if the joint movement previously was limited by soft tissue contracture. The main consistent postoperative outcome is pain relief.

Rough guidelines for return to functional activities are: driving, sedentary or light work, swimming, gardening (light) – 6–8 weeks; overhead activities/manual work – 3–6 months (perhaps never).

Most improvements are gained in the first 6 months, but improvements in strength and range of movement can continue for up to 18 months/2 years.

Manipulation under anaesthetic

These patients may be admitted overnight. They should be seen regularly by a physiotherapist during their stay. Outpatient physiotherapy needs to be implemented immediately to retain movement gained at operation.

Subacromial decompression

This operation is often done by arthroscopy. Although scars are small this operation can be very painful in the first few days as a result of bony resection and ligament release. Heavy lifting is discouraged in the first week, but otherwise patients are encouraged to regain their shoulder movements as soon as possible. This is not normally a problem. They can return to normal activities as they feel able, where possible avoiding shoulder impingement positions.

Rotator cuff repair

Although patients may only be in hospital for 1–3 days following this procedure, this operation can have a considerable rehabilitation period. The extent and security of the reconstruction can vary enormously and has a direct bearing on the rehabilitation times and outcomes. Patients may be immobilized for up to 6 weeks in a sling (and in some units a splint keeping the shoulder in abduction and external rotation). During this time the patients are normally given strict instructions on what to avoid and the joint may only be moved passively (no or minimal muscle contraction).

Once this initial period is over, the patient then embarks on a progressive exercise programme aimed to regain muscle control and range of movement. Supervised rehabilitation is vital for these patients.

General guidelines for return to functional activities are: driving – 5–9 weeks postoperatively; all lifting should be avoided for 3 months; patients with overhead or manual work may be off for 6 months.

Again the greatest progress is seen in the first 6 months, but improvements, particularly in strength, can continue for 2 years.

Elbow

General advice for elbow problems

- Local heat and/or cold may be helpful for pain relief (see Appendix 11.1 for details).
- Avoid repetitive wrist/forearm movements.
- If problems with sustained gripping activities, suggest change of grip size (e.g. enlarging diameter of pen size for writing) and also increase awareness to try and loosen grip to a minimum.

Elbow exercises

Many pains and discomforts around the elbow can be referred or influenced from the cervical spine. Worsening symptoms, particularly of paraesthesia, numbness or pain, should be viewed with caution and a reassessment of management made.

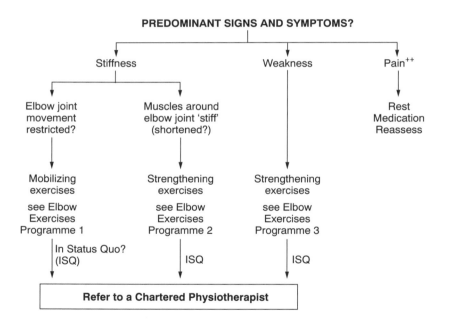

Elbow mobilizing exercises

Elbow Programme 1

Predominant signs and symptoms are of elbow joint stiffness.

Flexion (with supination)
Lying on back, upper arm supported on
bed/floor
Bend hand towards shoulder, palm facing
Then straighten arm out
Repeat 5–10 times

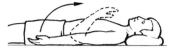

If weakness is not a problem this can be
done in standing or sitting

Can also add in forearm movements
Thumb towards shoulder (mid range)\
Back of hand towards shoulder (with
pronation)

Extension
In standing or lying
Keep elbow close to body
Straighten elbow as much as possible
(Can have palm facing in front, behind or
into body)
Repeat 5–10 times

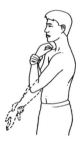

Supination
Standing or sitting
Elbow close to body and bent to 90 degrees
Turn forearm, so palm facing up to ceiling
Repeat 5–10 times
Can hold an end-weighted stick (e.g.
hammer) to add extra stretch

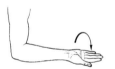

Pronation
As above but with facing down to floor
Also can add an end-weighted stick

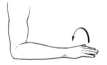

Elbow stretching exercises

Elbow Programme 2

Predominant signs and symptoms are of elbow stiffness related to shortened muscles.

Forearm extensors (i.e. tennis elbow)
Stand or sit
Straighten elbow (and keep it straight)
Curl fingers up into a fist
Then flex wrist
Hold for 20 seconds
Repeat 5 times

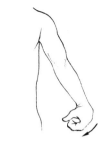

Forearm flexors (i.e. golfer's elbow)
Stand or sit
Link fingers together
Straighten elbow (and keep it straight)
Then extend wrist
Hold for 20 seconds
Repeat 5 times

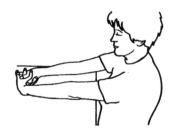

Elbow strengthening exercises

Elbow Programme 3
Predominant signs and symptoms are weakness of the elbow.

Extension (A)
Lying on stomach
Upper arm resting on bed
Straighten arm out
Repeat 20–30 times
Progress by adding weight in hand

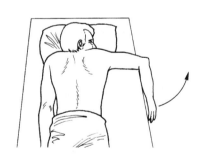

Extension (B)
Push-ups standing against wall
Progress to:
(a)   push-ups from knees
(b)   push-ups from toes
Repeat 10–20 times

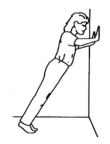

Flexion (and supination)
Stand or sit
Palm facing backwards
Bend elbow, palm towards shoulder
Repeat 20–30 times
Progress by adding weight in hand

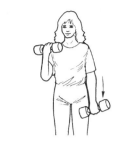

Pronation and supination (A)
Stand or sit
Elbow close to body and bent to 90 degree angle
Hold end-weighted stick (e.g. hammer)
Turn forearm so palm faces floor to ceiling
Keep control throughout the movement
Repeat 20–30 times

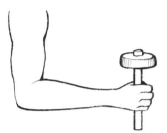

Pronation and supination (B)
Wringing action
Using a towel
Grip towel with hands
Twist arm in both directions
(palm up and palm down)

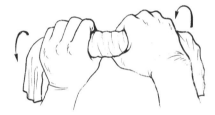

For forearm strengthening exercises, please see section on wrist strengthening exercises (Wrist Programme 2).

Postoperative management and advice

Total elbow replacement

The rehabilitation starts as inpatient, with input from both occupational therapists and physiotherapists. Assisted movements are commenced according to the surgeon's wishes (can start day 1 or not until day 3). Early mobilization is encouraged but the triceps repair needs protection for 6 weeks. Some centres use a removable posterior plaster of Paris shell during this period, others discharge the patients after approximately 10 days with a sling. Outpatient physiotherapy is normally arranged.

Patients can gradually increase their functional activities as able. Most patients with this operation have rheumatoid arthritis, and their functional ability after this operation may be influenced by their other joint problems. Pain relief is the prime aim of replacement and there is often a residual flexion deformity which does not normally interfere with function. The prostheses are not designed for heavy or high levels of activity, and these are generally discouraged.

Tennis elbow release

The exact surgical procedure may vary for this operation and postoperative rehabilitation will reflect this. Patients may attend as a day case and have no specific physiotherapy arranged (as in Oxford), whereas others can have the elbow immobilized for 2 weeks and then follow a full rehabilitation programme over 8 weeks. Forearm support bands can continue to be used for working/leisure activities to reduce the possibility of recurrence.

Wrist and hand

The exercises presented here are mainly for the wrist. The hand tends to exercise itself with everyday use. Following injury or trauma, especially involving damage to tendon or nerve, the hand requires specific rehabilitation under the supervision of surgeon and therapy staff. Therefore hand exercises, other than general grip strengthening, have not been included. Giving advice on joint protection strategies however can be of considerable benefit to those with degenerative joint disease of the wrist and hand, and some ideas are given. For more detailed advice and assessment refer to hand or occupational therapist.

General advice and strategies for joint protection of the hand (e.g. thumb carpometacarpal (CMC) and metacarpophalangeal (MCP) joints, OA or RA)

- Use tap turners (variety of models), electrical tin openers.
- When sustained gripping required, enlarge grip size to change the loading on the joints (e.g. on tools, pens, kitchen items).
- Local warmth may be helpful for pain relief. Warm water can be used. More heat can be given to the joint if rubber gloves protect the skin (see Appendix 11.1).
- If the hand feels weak, advise patient to try exercising (general gripping action) against spongy material e.g. Childrens Play Doh or can make their own using 1 cup of water, 1 cup of flour, 1/2 cup of salt, 1 tablespoon of cooking oil, 1 teaspoon of cream of tartar, food colouring. Boil these together and keep in polythene bag. The putty can be used without taking it out of the bag.

General advice for people with wrist problems

- Local heat and/or cold may be helpful for pain relief (see Appendix 11.1 for details).

- Wrist supports may be helpful (with the wrist held in some extension). Advise intermittent use at night (e.g. carpal tunnel) or during day (when involved in gripping or lifting activities). NB: Patients with De Quervain's tendonitis require thumb immobilization as well.

Wrist exercises

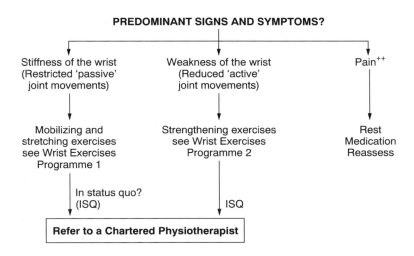

PREDOMINANT SIGNS AND SYMPTOMS?

Stiffness of the wrist (Restricted 'passive' joint movements)	Weakness of the wrist (Reduced 'active' joint movements)	Pain[++]
Mobilizing and stretching exercises see Wrist Exercises Programme 1	Strengthening exercises see Wrist Exercises Programme 2	Rest Medication Reassess
In status quo? (ISQ)	ISQ	

Refer to a Chartered Physiotherapist

Mobilizing exercises for the wrist

Wrist Programme 1

Predominant signs and symptoms are of stiffness in wrist.
There is some overlap between the exercises for the elbow and wrist.

Advice: These exercises may be more comfortable after the application of local heat.

Extension (A)
Place hand and forearm flat on table/surface
Lift hand up in air
Keep forearm down
Repeat 5–10 times
NB: If elbow extension is maintained throughout, the forearm flexors will be stretched

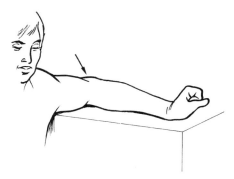

Extension (B)

Place elbows and palms of hands together
in front of body
Keep palms together
Take elbows apart
Repeat 5–10 times

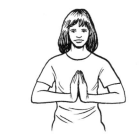

Flexion

Place forearms on table, palm down
Place wrist crease on edge of table
Let hand drop over edge of table
Can add a stretch with other hand
Repeat 5–10 times
NB: If elbow extension is maintained
throughout, the forearm extensors will be
stretched

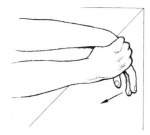

Radial and ulnar deviation

Place forearm and hand on table, palm
down
Keep forearm still
Slide hand from one side to other side
Repeat 5–10 times each side

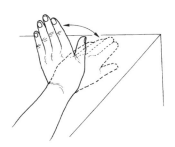

Supination and pronation

See elbow exercises for description of exercises

Strengthening exercises for the wrist

Wrist Programme 2

The predominant signs and symptoms are of weakness of the wrist.

Forearm extensors

Forearm resting on table, palm down
Wrist crease on edge of table, hand dropped
over edge of table
Lift hand up
Repeat 20–30 times
Progress by:
(i)   adding ulnar and radial deviation
(ii) holding a weight
(iii) pulling against an elastic rope

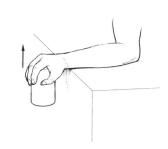

188

Forearm flexors
Forearm resting on table, palm facing up
Wrist crease on edge of table, hand dropped
over edge
Lift hand up
Repeat 20–30 times
Progress by:

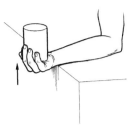

(i)   adding ulnar and radial deviation
(ii) holding a weight
(iii) pulling against an elastic rope

Postoperative management and advice

Carpal tunnel release

This procedure is done as a day case. Patients are discharged with a bulky bandage, maintained for 2 weeks. They are encouraged to resume daily activities as able and will not have outpatient physiotherapy arranged, unless they are experiencing problems in regaining function.

Guidelines for return to activities are: return to light work within 3 to 4 weeks; return to heavy work between 8 and 12 weeks; grip strength and endurance may take 3–6 months or longer to achieve, And for some may remain incomplete.

Surgical release of Dupytren's contracture

This procedure is also done as a day case. Patients will be discharged with a plaster of Paris backslab and bulky bandage which is maintained for 2–3 days (longer if a skin graft has been taken). If no skin graft is taken, patients are seen by a hand therapist around the third postoperative day to remove the bandage, commence mobilization and to fit a splint. The splint is used to counteract the tendency for the surgical scar to contract during wound healing. Most patients wear the splint at night for 3 months (or longer) and some wear it during the day as well.

Therapy aims to maintain the finger extension range gained from surgery and to restore preoperative flexion. In a few cases specific treatment modalities are required, for example, ultrasound, serial splinting, silicone elastomere treatment.

Guidelines for return to functional activities are: return to desk job – 2–6 weeks; return to driving – 2–4 weeks; return to manual work – 6–8 weeks.

Cervical spine

Neck pain and related symptoms into the arm, shoulder and head can be very frightening for patients and may lead to patterns of disability similar to those described by the Clinical Standards Advisory Group on back pain (Clinical Standards Advisory Group, 1994). Therefore reassurance combined with practical advice and early active treatment, particularly for patients who appear anxious or distressed, is advised.

General advice for people with cervical spine problems

- Give them confidence and positive reassurance of the body's ability to heal, but it does require an encouraging environment!
- Patients should be encouraged to remain active, with activities that do not worsen the pain. This can be more difficult than for lumbar spine pain. Jolting movements often hurt (wear soft-soled shoes/walk on flat surfaces) and swimming and cycling can result in painful sustained neck postures unless patients are specifically advised to change their head/body position regularly.
- Be aware of language/labels and their possible effects (e.g. arthritis of the spine or whiplash) which may be frightening to patients and increase disability (e.g. a common thought is 'Dr says it is "wearing out" therefore I must use it less').
- Unloading the compressive force through the spine can be helpful. Advise patients to use resting positions in lying, with the head supported with pillows so that it is comfortable. This can be no pillows for some, but often those with nerve root symptoms prefer two or more.
- Collars can be helpful, particularly with early-onset, severe pain and if a patient is finding it difficult to hold their head up. Following whiplash-type injuries, collars holding the head in slight flexion may be more comfortable. However, continuous and prolonged use of a collar should be discouraged and is associated with a poor prognosis following whiplash injuries. Promote intermittent use. Soft collars worn at night may be helpful. Collars can disturb balance for some patients and wearing one as a driver can be awkward, requires adaptation (use of mirrors) and may have implications for their car insurance policy.
- When sitting it may be more comfortable to lean back and have the head and neck supported. If the patient is still very uncomfortable, it is advisable to lie down. If sitting at a workstation or watching television, suggest the screen is straight ahead and make sure the **lumbar** spine is straight or in lordosis (use rolled-up towel or cushion, etc.; see lumbar spine advice below).
- Avoid sustained stooping postures and sitting or standing with the head forwards and unsupported.
- Attention to the pillow arrangement is indicated if the pain is worse at night or on waking. The depth of pillow should be that of the distance from the shoulder to the side of the head. To support the neck, a rolled-up hand towel (or roll of foam) can be placed down the front of the pillowcase to give extra support (Figure 11.7). This works best with a soft top pillow.

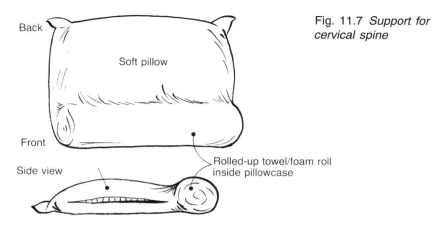

Fig. 11.7 *Support for cervical spine*

- Avoiding sleeping on the stomach may also reduce symptoms.
- Heat pads or hot water bottles can be helpful on overactive muscles (often upper trapezius). Cold (ice) packs can also be tried and local massage.
- Reduce stress levels as much as possible with use of music, relaxation tapes, etc.

Cervical spine exercises

With cervical spine exercises, pain/paraesthesia **should not peripheralize**, i.e. pain becomes more prominent away from the cervical area (into head, scapula, shoulders, arm and/or hands), even if the cervical pain is resolving. With peripheral signs and symptoms, cervical spine pain can worsen **as long as peripheral symptoms are easing**. If the patient has arm pain, check the neurological signs and always heed these precautions. If the exercise does not relieve the pain (in the manner stated above), advise patients to discontinue that particular exercise, but continue with others and general advice strategies.

Cervical spine presentations have been divided grossly into two categories. First those with localized neck pain, secondly those with referred pain into the head, scapula, shoulder or arm. The presentations can be extremely varied in terms of severity and irritability (e.g. how easy to exacerbate symptoms and how long to settle), and to reflect this they have been further divided.

Moderate or severe nerve root pain requires individual assessment and treatment with close monitoring of neurological signs and symptoms. For those with mild symptoms, the exercises can be tried but the warnings/precautions must be given. Be cautious of patients who present with minimal or moderate symptoms but whose head and shoulders are in abnormal postures (e.g. head sideflexed and/or rotated). The postures are commonly antalgic and movements reversing them can significantly worsen symptoms. Refer these cases to a chartered physiotherapist for individual assessment.

The exercise programmes have not been subdivided into flexion/extension patterns as combined movements are used. Commonly the cervical spine is in an overused posture of upper cervical extension and lower cervical flexion (i.e. chin poke with cervicothoracic kyphosis) and this can be regarded as the equivalent to 'slumped' posture of the lumbar spine. In fact the two postures are inter-related.

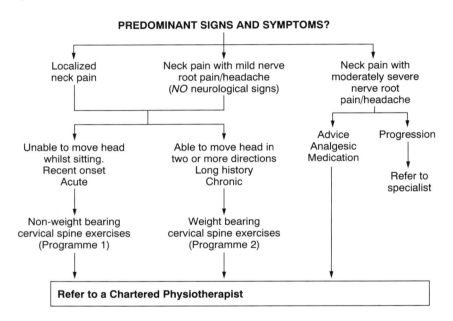

Cervical Spine Programme 1

The predominant symptoms are local cervical spine pain and/or mild arm symptoms without neurological changes with **recent onset symptoms (i.e. 'acute')**. The patient may have severe limitation of movement (only move in one or two directions) in sitting or standing (antigravity postures).

NB: All these exercises are designed to try and relieve pain. Pain must either ease with repetition, stay the same, or move up the arm towards the cervical spine. It must not get worse or move into the head, arm (and scapula).

If the exercise does not relieve the pain (in the manner stated above), advise patients to discontinue that particular exercise, but continue with others and general advice strategies.

Non-weightbearing exercises
- These exercises should be done in a pain-free starting position if possible.
- This may require one or more pillows which can be gradually reduced until the head is resting on the floor/bed.
- A heat pad can also be used at the same time (hot water bottle half full).
- The exercises can be done 20–30 minutes after appropriate medication.

Shoulder shrug in lying
Gently raise shoulders up towards ears
Try and get both sides to move
smoothly
Then let them relax
Repeat 5–10 times

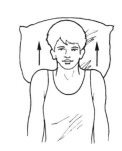

Upper cervical flexion, lower cervical extension in lying
Keep head *supported* on pillow/floor
throughout the movement
Tuck chin in
Pressing back of neck towards
pillow/floor
It is like a small nodding movement
A stretch is normally felt at the back of
the neck
(Do not clench teeth during this)
Repeat 5–10 times

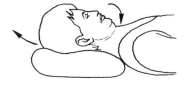

Cervical rotations in lying
Keep head *supported* on pillow/floor
throughout the movement
Try and keep chin tucked in as in
exercise above
Turn head, so looking to side
Return to midline
Repeat 5 times to one side, then repeat
to other side

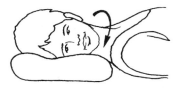

(Can progress onto Cervical Spine Programme 2 if symptoms settle)

Cervical Spine Programme 2

Exercises for patients with local cervical spine pain and/or mild arm symptoms without neurological changes with **insiduous onset and long-term symptoms (i.e. 'chronic')**. Only one or two movement directions may be limited.

NB: All these exercises are designed to try and relieve pain. Pain must either ease with repetition, stay the same, or move up the arm towards the cervical spine. It must not get worse or move into the head, arm (and scapula).

If the exercise does not relieve the pain (in the manner stated above), advise patients to discontinue that particular exercise, but continue with others and general advice strategies.

Weightbearing exercises
If the patient is unable to do these, go to Cervical Spine Programme 1.

Upper cervical flexion, lower cervical extension in sitting
Sitting in a firm (and high) backed chair
Look straight ahead
Pull chin in
Lift crown of head up
Feel stretch at back of neck
Do not let chin drop down (so head is forward)
Repeat 5–10 times
Can start this:
(i)   sitting with back and head resting against wall/back of door
(ii) if pain is unilateral try with head slightly tilted (side flexed) to one side

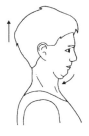

Upper cervical flexion, lower cervical extension in sitting with overpressure
Sitting in a firm (and high) backed chair
Repeat exercise as above
Put hands on chin
Push chin further backwards
Hold for 5 seconds
Repeat 5–10 times

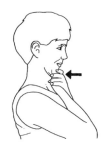

Cervical rotation (discontinue if dizzy or lightheaded)
Sitting upright
Try and keep chin gently pulled in (as above)
Turn head to one side
Aim to get chin over shoulder
Repeat 5 times to one side, then repeat to other side

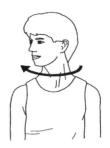

Cervical side flexion (discontinue if dizzy or lightheaded)
Sitting upright
Try and keep chin gently pulled in (as above)
Look straight ahead
Tilt ear towards shoulder
(Often will feel stretch on opposite side)
Repeat 5 time to one side, then repeat to other side

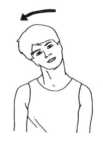

Cervical extension (discontinue if dizzy or lightheaded)
Sitting upright
Do first exercise in this programme
Then at finishing point, look up at ceiling
Starting by giving support at back of head with fingers
Try and keep chin tucked in on return to starting position
Repeat 5–10 times

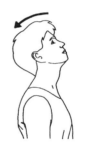

Cervical traction
Sitting upright
Place clenched fist between chin and chest
Put other hand behind head
Gently pull head forward and down
Feel stretch at back of neck
Repeat 5–10 times

(May need to put a book or folded towel under clenched hand to affect the upper cervical spine)

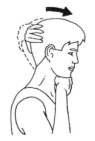

Postoperative management and advice

Anterior cervical decompression and fusion

This operation may be performed by either an orthopaedic surgeon or neurosurgeon. The use of collars routinely in postoperative care has not been established. They may not be given at all or given for comfort, intermittent use or for more consistent use. Therefore check local protocols. Firm or soft collars can be used during the day (e.g. travelling), with a soft collar used at night. Outpatient physiotherapy may not be instigated, with patients given encouragement by the surgeons and staff to regain neck movements and general activities gradually. Neck movements should be re-established within 3 months, with minimal restriction for those who have had a single-level fusion. Often, however, it is arm pain, sensory changes and motor weakness in arms and/or legs that are of prime concern in terms of outcome. However, if a patient appears to be very frightened regarding neck movements and does not appear to be progressing with self-directed rehabilitation, consider referral to physiotherapy.

Guidelines for return to functional activities are: return to light work – 4–6 weeks; return to driving – 4–6 weeks unless hard collar is worn (see previous advice on collar and driving); avoid lifting completely for 6 weeks and then start with light items; return to heavy work – 6–12 weeks.

Lumbar spine

General advice for people with lumbar spine problems

- Give them confidence and positive reassurance of natural history and that the back has a good ability to heal, given an encouraging environment.
- Beware of using frightening language/labels such as 'arthritis of the spine'.
- Patients should be encouraged to remain active, with activities that do not worsen the pain.
- Unloading the compression force through the spine can be helpful as in lying and swimming, but *prolonged bed rest* (over 3 days for simple backache, 2 weeks for nerve root pain) is *not* advised.
- Sitting is often problematical except for the patients with spinal stenosis. Advise patients to avoid sitting as much as possible, and to lie, stand or walk. When sitting, they are often more comfortable when they have increased lumbar lordosis (not slumping). This can be achieved by perching on edge of seats/chairs and by placing a rolled-up towel or cushion in the small of their back or using a wedge

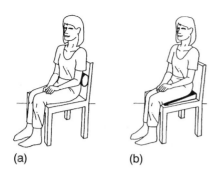

Fig. 11.10 *a, Sitting postures: using a lumbar 'roll'; b, sitting postures: using a wedge*

(a)   (b)

(Figure 11.10). The car seat often presents problems; use a roll and try taking the seat towards steering wheel as well.
- Avoid sustained stooping postures and lifting.
- Firm up soft mattresses/beds. Try a rolled-up towel in the waist (like a lifebuoy, and/or pillow between the legs if having problems getting comfortable at night).
- Use heat or cold on the area or local massage for pain relief.
- Reduce stress levels as much as possible with use of music, relaxation tapes, etc.
- This position (Figure 11.11: Fowler's resting position) is often helpful. It places the spine in a neutral, unloaded position.

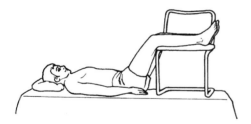

Fig. 11.11 *Fowler's resting position*

Written advice in the form of a booklet was shown to have a positive effect on patients presenting with lower back pain in general practice. This booklet is now in the process of being updated by a multidisciplinary group of clinicians and researchers in conjunction with the Department of Health. It is available from HMSO (1996).

Lumbar spine exercises

- As recommended by the Clinical Standards Advisory Group (1994), the category of mechanical low back pain can be divided into simple backache and nerve root pain (see Lumbar Spine chapter for clinical criteria). These exercises can be applied to patients with simple backache and those with mild nerve root pain. If they have leg pain, check the neurological signs and always heed these precautions.

- **Pain should not progressively worsen, during or after these exercises. In particular, pain should not peripheralize (i.e. increasing pain in buttocks, leg, ankle or foot with lumbar spine pain). If there are peripheral pain symptoms, lumbar spine pain can worsen as long as the peripheral symptoms are easing.**
- People in distress with their problem, or those with nerve root signs, may require early referral to a chartered physiotherapist for an individual assessment.

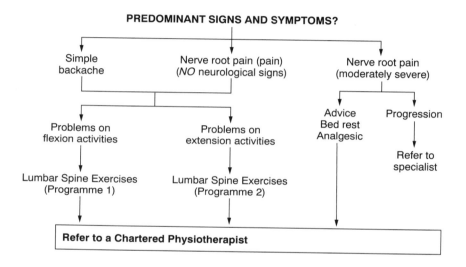

Lumbar Spine Programme 1

For patients with simple backache and/or mild leg pain without neurological changes with problems mainly on flexion (and sitting) (e.g. cannot flex forward to get shoes/socks/clothes on, worse sitting slumped, driving, stooping activities, lifting).

NB: All these exercises are designed to try and relieve pain. Pain must either ease with repetition, stay the same, or move up the leg/limb towards the lumbar spine. It must not get worse or move down the leg.

If the exercise does not relieve the pain (in the manner stated above), advise patients to discontinue that particular exercise, but continue with others and general advice strategies.

If hips are shifted over to one side, or pain is unilateral, try side glides first. If this is not so, go to next exercise.

Side glides in standing

Try this initially moving hips in the *opposite direction* to where they are shifted
Stand sideways, with shoulder and arm against wall, elbow bent
Feet about 10 cm away from the wall
Move hips sideways towards the wall
Hold for 5 seconds
Repeat 10 times

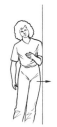

Passive extension in prone lying

If the patient is unable to tolerate this, can start with simple lying with pillows under hips/lower abdomen
Lying on stomach
Hands under shoulder as if doing a press up
Keep back muscles relaxed
Push through arms, straightening elbows
Keep the hips and pelvis down
Feel back arching
Breathe out to get extra stretch
Repeat 10 times regularly (e.g. 2 hourly or more)

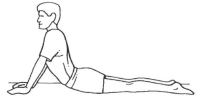

Extension in standing

Standing with your hands on your hips
Keep knees straight
Lean back
Do not let hips move forwards
Repeat 10 times regularly
(This may not be as effective as relieving pain as the exercise in lying, but it may be easier to do in everyday life).

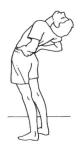

Lumbar Spine Programme 2

For patients with simple backache and/or mild leg pain without neuro-logical changes with problems on extension activities (e.g. swimming on stomach, lying on stomach, walking, returning to upright position from being bent over, sit to standing, reaching up, wearing high heels). NB: These patients are different to those who are 'stuck' in flexion, often with nerve root pain, who may respond to the exercises in Programme 1.

NB: All these exercises are designed to try and relieve pain. Pain must either ease with repetition, stay the same, or move up the leg/limb towards the lumbar spine. It must not get worse or move down the leg.

If the exercise does not relieve the pain (in the manner stated above), advise patients to discontinue that particular exercise, but continue with others and general advice strategies.

Flexion in lying
Lying on back
Take one knee up onto chest
Hug it with arms, pulling knee
up towards nose
Repeat with other knee
Try with both knees to chest
Repeat 10 times

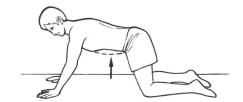

Abdominals in prone kneeling
On all fours, with back straight
Pull *low* tummy in
Try and flatten it
Breathe easily
Hold for 20–30 seconds

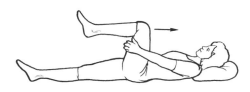

Flexion and extension in prone kneeling
On all fours
Tighten stomach muscles to
flex or 'round' back
Then let back extend or
'hollow'
Keep elbows straight and arms
still
Repeat 10 times

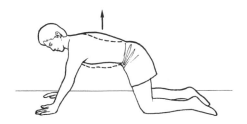

Flexion in prone kneeling
On all fours
Keep hands stretched out in
front
Sit back on heels
Let shoulders lower towards
floor/bed
Hold for 5 seconds
Repeat 5 times

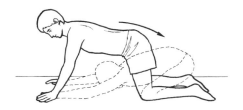

Flexion in crook lying
Lie with knees bent, feet flat
on floor/bed
Tighten low stomach muscles
(flatten them)
Try and press back into
floor/bed
Do not use feet to push!
Hold for 20 seconds, breathe
easily
Repeat 10–15 times

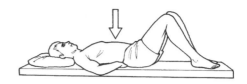

Flexion in standing
Stand with back against wall
Heels 10 cm away
Feet shoulder width apart
Tighten low stomach muscles
Try and move low back so it is
touching the wall
Repeat 10 times

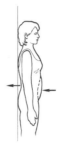

Postoperative management and advice

Lumbar surgery may be undertaken by either a neurosurgeon or orthopaedic surgeon. This may also introduce a further variable to the postoperative management.

Lumbar discectomy

This operation is becoming less invasive (micro-discectomy), resulting in shorter inpatient stays and quicker rehabilitation. The following guidelines refer to a traditional discectomy protocol. Patients may have been seen by a physiotherapist (and possibly an occupational therapist) whilst in hospital and given advice, education and a simple home exercise programme.

Generally activity is encouraged. For example, walking as much as possible, increasing the distance covered. Swimming may be started once the wound is healed. Sitting is often restricted (due to the intradiscal pressure). Patients may be advised to perch, sit in higher chairs and use a cushion, towel or roll of foam in their low back. Prolonged sitting is discouraged (i.e. 20–30 minutes maximum by 2 weeks) and active strategies must be adopted to avoid 'slumping' (i.e. changing chairs, using extra supports, etc.). Driving may not be possible for 6 weeks and is dependent on sitting tolerance and the pain response and flexibility of knee extension in sitting. Lifting is restricted commonly for several weeks (e.g. 8–12 weeks), and for those unable to avoid it altogether (i.e. those with small children), guidelines should have been given regarding lifting techniques (keep objects close being the most important). Outpatient physiotherapy appointments may be made by the hospital staff on discharge or this may be initiated by the doctors when the patient is reviewed in an outpatient clinic. Routine outpatient physiotherapy may not be given. If a patient appears to be distressed or not gradually regaining activity, seek advice from the hospital (surgeon or physiotherapist), who may suggest that referral to a physiotherapist is indicated to supervise rehabilitation.

Lumbar decompression

The surgery involved in this procedure can vary considerably in its extent of bony resection. Rehabilitation may reflect this. Generally the principles of early mobilization and improving general fitness will be followed as with the discectomies. Greater emphasis may be placed on abdominal control and lumbar flexion range. Milestones of return to functional activities are as for patients following discectomy.

Spinal fusion

The postoperative care of these patients is similar to other spinal surgery as above, but spinal movements are not encouraged excessively during the first 3 months of rehabilitation whilst the bone grafts are healing and the fusion is not biologically sound. The home exercise programme will emphasize muscle stabilizing work (abdominals, deep back extensors and gluteals).

Lifting should be avoided for the first 3 months and restriction on sitting (see Lumbar Discectomy above) is also advised. However walking and swimming can be encouraged as above.

Outpatient physiotherapy to progress the exercise programme may be organized for 6 weeks or thereafter by hospital staff or doctors in outpatient clinics.

Chemonucleolysis

This operation involves an injection of an enzyme (chymopapain) into the nucleus of the disc in the treatment of a disc prolapse (if the disc is not sequestrated). It is normally done as day surgery. Again prolonged sitting and lifting are not encouraged, particularly in the first 6 weeks.

Hip

General advice for people with hip problems

- Keep the joint moving but without stressing it, e.g. avoid unnecessary lifting, stairs, squat, twisting and turning activities.
- Try swimming or movements in water.
- Try static cycling (seat may need to be raised).
- Raise seat heights and when getting out of chairs, use hands to push up with.
- Use a walking aid (stick or crutches) if unable to put all the weight through leg. Use a stick in the **opposite** hand. Try and walk as normally as possible with the walking aid.

Hip exercises

Be aware that buttock pain can be referred from the lumbar spine.

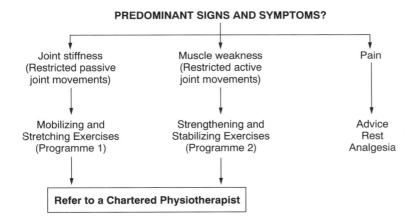

PREDOMINANT SIGNS AND SYMPTOMS?

Joint stiffness (Restricted passive joint movements) → Mobilizing and Stretching Exercises (Programme 1)

Muscle weakness (Restricted active joint movements) → Strengthening and Stabilizing Exercises (Programme 2)

Pain → Advice Rest Analgesia

Refer to a Chartered Physiotherapist

Hip mobilizing exercises

Hip Programme 1

For predominant signs and symptoms of stiffness of the hip joint.

Advice: It may be useful to do these after application of local heat (e.g. warm bath/shower, see Appendix 11.1).

Hip flexion in lying
Lying on back, legs out
straight
Bend knee up towards chest
Return to start position
Repeat 5–10 times

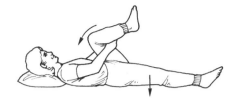

Hip flexion in standing
Stand facing a step (book or
telephone directory if step is
too high)
Place foot up onto step
Keep trunk still
Return to starting position
Gradually place foot on higher
surface (use a stool/chair)
Repeat 5–10 times

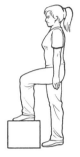

Hip extension in lying
Bend both knees up towards
chest
Hug *unaffected* knee with
hands (keep the pressure on)
Straighten out affected leg
May feel stretch in front of hip
This can be done on edge of
table/bed to get more stretch
Repeat 5 times

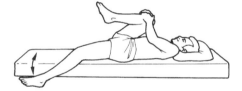

Hip extension in prone lying
Lie on stomach
Try and get front of hips in
contact with bed/floor (may
need to start with small pillow
or towel)
Tighten buttock muscles
Hold for 10 seconds
Repeat 10 times
(i)   Try and rest in this
position for 15–20 seconds
(ii)   Try and bend knee,
keeping hips down into
bed/floor
(iii)   Can then add knee lift
(see Hip Programme 2)

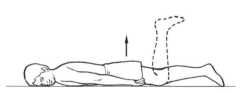

Medial rotation in prone lying
Lie on stomach
Bend knee to 90 degree angle
Keep knee still but let foot fall
out to side (away from other
leg)
Repeat 5–10 times

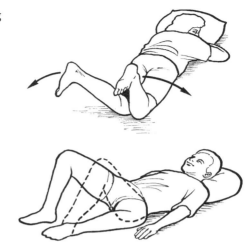

**Abduction and external
rotation**
Lie on back, knees bent up,
feet on bed/floor
Let knees separate, keeping
feet together
Do not let back arch
Repeat 5–10 times

Hip strengthening exercises

Hip Programme 2

For predominant signs and symptoms of weakness and instability
around the hip joint.

Where possible use the weightbearing exercises as they are more
functionally relevant and easier to practice!

Non-weightbearing exercises
Bridging
Lie on back, knee bent up, feet
on bed/floor
Flatten back towards bed/floor
Lift buttocks off the bed/floor
Repeat 20–30 times
Progress to:
(i)   lifting *unaffected* other foot
off bed/floor
(ii)·   pushing up through
affected leg alone

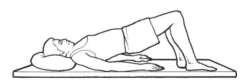

Extension in prone lying
Lying on stomach, knee bent to
90 degree angle
Lift knee 1 cm off bed/floor
Do not let back overarch
Repeat 20–30 times
NB: if unable to do this start
with knee straight

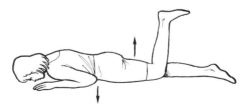

205

Weightbearing exercises
Sit to standing

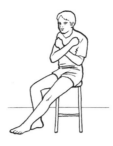
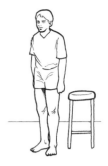

Sit on high surface (stool or arm
of sofa or armchair)
Keep affected leg back, other leg
slightly forward
Cross arms and try and stand up
Then sit down slowly
Repeat 20–30 times
Progress by lowering the height
of the seat to a normal chair
Further progress by lifting
unaffected leg off ground

Step ups

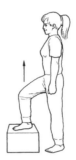

Step up onto a step using affected
leg
Start with a small step (e.g.
telephone directory)
Gradually increase depth of step
Repeat (aim for) 20–30 times

Dynamic alignment work in standing

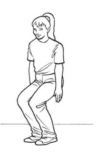

This aims to retrain muscle control
and balance. It may also stretch
the calf
Stand with feet hip width apart
Keep body upright
Bend knees fairly slowly, making
sure knees are moving over
second toe
Keep heels on the ground
Start with small dips and increase
gradually (without pain)
Repeat 10–15 times, once a day
minimum
Progress further by:
(i)   doing on one leg,
maintaining balance
(ii)   stepping down off a small
step (heel will come off ground
for this)
(iii) increase the depth of the step

Balance
Practice standing on one leg
Progress by a) closing eyes b) onto
tiptoe

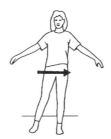

Postoperative management and advice

Total hip replacement

These patients are commonly in hospital for 10 days. Most hip replacements are cemented and patients can weightbear as tolerated and leave hospital when at a safe, functional level with a good gait pattern using crutches or two sticks. Patients are assessed by the occupational therapy team and given seat raises, helping hands (to avoid bending to floor level) and bath boards as necessary. They are not normally given outpatient physiotherapy appointments, but encouraged to increase their activity level as able.

Precautions need to be taken for the first 3 months. Patients should avoid hip flexion (over 90 degree angle), particularly combined with adduction (e.g. sitting crossed legged, bending forward and lying on their non-operated side with the top leg unsupported). Patients are advised to sleep on their backs with a pillow between their legs for 6 weeks, after which time they can lie as they find comfortable.

Other than these restrictions, patients are encouraged to gradually increase their activity, especially walking. If the patient continues to have a poor gait pattern, referral to physiotherapy may be indicated. Poor gait is often due to disuse atrophy of the gluteals muscles and may require strengthening work (see strengthening exercises: Hip Programme 2).

Guidelines for return to other functional activities are: driving – after 6–8 weeks; return to desk job – after 6–10 weeks; return to manual work – 6 months, possibly never; swimming can be started as soon as the wound is healed but breast stroke should be avoided for the first 6 weeks; cycling can commence once sufficient range of motion is available, but the seat may need to be raised so that the hip is not flexing over 90 degrees; gardening may not be possible for 3–4 months. Patients with uncemented hip replacements may have restricted weightbearing for 6–12 weeks but otherwise follow a similar (but slower) postoperative regime as described above.

There is now a booklet (Total Hip Replacement 'Information for Patients') available nationally for patients having, or likely to have, total hip replacements from the Royal College of Surgeons, Audit Department (if sponsorship has been re-secured.) The postage costs need to be paid, but otherwise it is free and it covers the preoperative, operative and postoperative process.

Knee

General advice for people with knee problems

- Avoid activities which increase swelling and/or pain. (Swelling will result in reflex inhibition of quadriceps, irrespective of the presence of pain.)
- Keep the joint moving but without stressing it, e.g. avoid unnecessary lifting, stairs, squat, kneeling, uneven ground, twisting and turning activities.
- Try static cycling (put the seat up high if movement is limited).
- Try swimming (freestyle legs may be more comfortable than breast stroke legs if there is instability).
- Local heat and/or cold may be helpful (see Appendix 11.1 for details).
- Raise seat heights and use hands to push up with when getting out of chairs.
- Use a walking aid (stick or crutches) if unable to put all the weight through the leg. Use a stick in the **opposite** hand. Try and walk as normally as possible with the walking aid.

Knee exercises

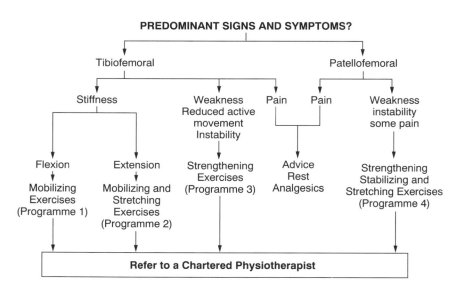

Knee mobilizing exercises (tibiofemoral joint)

Knee Programme 1

For patients with predominant signs and symptoms of **stiffness** of the tibiofemoral joint into **flexion**.

Knee flexion in sitting

Sit on a chair/table so you can
get foot underneath
Bend knee, taking foot under
chair as far as possible
Straighten knee out
Start with a small range of
movement and gradually
increase
Repeat 5–10 times

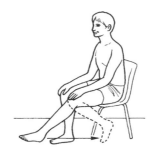

Knee flexion in prone lying

Lying on stomach, legs
together
Bend knee as far as possible
Do not let hips rise
May feel stretch in front of
thigh or hip
Can give overpressure using
the other leg
Repeat 5–10 times

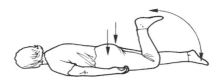

Knee Programme 2

For patients with predominant signs and symptoms of **stiffness** of tibiofemoral joint into **extension**.

Knee extension in sitting

Sit on a chair/table
Lean back, recline
Straighten knee out as far as
possible
Start with a small range of
movement and gradually
increase
Repeat 5–10 times

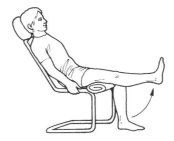

Knee extension in sitting/lying

Sit leaning back or lie on back
with leg supported
Place small towel under heel
Let gravity stretch joint into
extension
Can add hand pressure to give
extra stretch
Try and rest in this position for
several minutes
Increases to 10–15 minutes

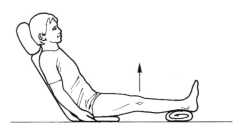

Knee strengthening exercises (tibiofemoral joint)

Knee Programme 3

For patients with predominant signs and symptoms of **weakness and
instability**.

NB: Straight-leg raising is not helpful, it mainly exercises the hip flexors!

The programme is divided into weightbearing and non-weightbearing
exercises. Weightbearing exercises should be used as long as there is no
increase in pain or swelling, as they are more functionally relevant and
easy to practice in everyday life.

Non-weightbearing exercises
Static quadriceps

If unable to do this try inner
range exercise
Half lying (e.g. propped up on
elbow)
Pull foot up
Push knee down into
bed/floor
Try and raise heel (but keep
knee down)
Hold for 5 seconds and relax
Repeat or aim for 20–30 times

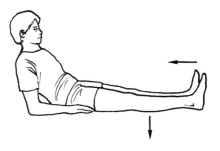

Inner range quadriceps

Half lying (propped up)
Rolled-up towel under knee
Pull toes up towards you
Straighten leg
Keep knee down on towel
Hold for 5 seconds
Repeat (aim for) 20–30 times

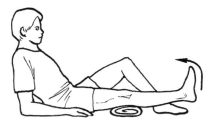

Static quadriceps/gluteals/adductors

Sitting with folded pillow or football between knees
Feet flat on ground
Knees bent *less than* 90 degrees
Squeeze knees together (into pillow/football)
Push feet into ground and away from body
Feel and see thigh muscles tighten
Hold for 5 seconds
Repeat 20–30 times
Progress by *adding*:
(i)   buttock squeeze
(ii)   lift opposite buttock off chair

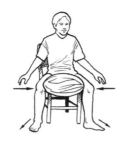

Weightbearing exercises

These **must** be painfree and not result in increased swelling.

Sit to standing

Sit on a high surface (stool or arm of sofa or armchair)
Keep affected leg back, other leg slightly forward
Cross arms and try and stand up
Then sit down slowly
Repeat (aim for) 20–30 times
Progress by lowering height of seat to a normal chair
Further progress by lifting unaffected leg off ground

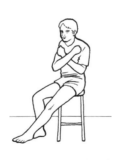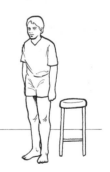

Step ups

Step up onto a step using affected leg
Start with a small step (e.g. telephone directory)
Gradually increase depth of step
Repeat (aim for) 20–30 times

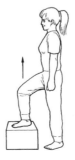

Dynamic alignment work in standing

This aims to retain muscle control and
balance. It may also stretch the calf
Stand with feet hip-width apart
Keep body upright
Bend knees fairly slowly, making sure knees
are moving over second toe. When looking
down inside knees, big toes should be seen
Keep heels on the ground
Start with small dips and increase gradually
(without pain)
Repeat 10–15 times, once a day minimum
Progress further by:
(i)   doing on one leg, maintaining balance
(ii)   stepping down off a small step (heel
will come off ground for this)
(iii)   increase depth of the step

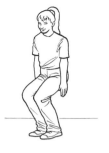

Hamstring strength and proprioception

Standing, hold on for support
Bend knee, lifting heel towards buttocks
Move it over a small distance, up and down
Then stop it suddenly
Repeat in different amounts of knee bend
Progress by adding weight at ankle
Repeat (aim for) 3–10 sets of 10 repetitions
or until fatigue

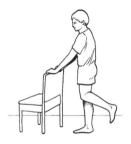

Balance

Practice standing on one leg
Progress onto tip-toe
Repeat with:
(i)   eyes closed
(ii)   on tiptoes

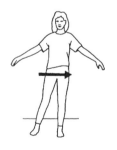

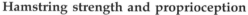

Exercises for patellofemoral symptoms

Knee Programme 4

Advice: Avoid squatting down and sustained weightbearing activities
on a bent knee.

Give stretches if muscles shortened on symptomatic side, otherwise start
on dynamic alignment exercise and sitting against the wall.

**NB: These exercises should be painfree, but may feel tight, stretched,
tired or wobbly.**

Non-weightbearing exercises
Static quadriceps/gluteals/adductors
Sitting with folded pillow or football
between knees
Feet flat on ground
Knees bent *less than* 90 degrees
Squeeze knees together (into
pillow/football)
Push feet into ground and away from body
Feel and see thigh muscles tighten
Hold for 5 seconds
Repeat 20–30 times
Progress by *adding*:
(i)   buttock squeeze
(ii) lift opposite buttock off chair

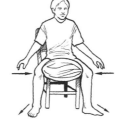

Weightbearing exercises
Dynamic alignment work in standing
(This aims to retain muscle control and
balance. It may also stretch the calf)
Stand with feet hip width apart
Keep body upright
Bend knees fairly slowly, making sure knees
are moving over second toe. When looking
down inside knees, big toes should be seen
Keep heels on the ground
Start with small dips and increase gradually
(without pain)
Repeat 10–15 times, once a day minimum
Progress further by:
(i)   doing on one leg, maintaining balance
(ii) stepping down off a small step (heel
will come off ground for this)
(iii) increase depth of the step

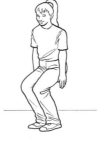

Sit against wall
Stand with back and heels against wall
Take three heel to toe steps forward,
keeping back against wall (this is important)
Slide back down wall, so sitting with knees
at approximately 60 degrees off full
extension
Hold for 10 seconds
Repeat 10–20 times
Then try and maintain position for 3
minutes

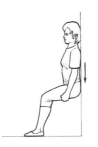

Hamstring stretches

NB: if symptoms of pain or paraesthesiae occur into calf/foot, discontinue and reassess
Lying on back
Link arms around back of thigh
Straighten knee
Feel pull in back of thigh, buttock or knee
Hold for 20 seconds, repeat 5 times

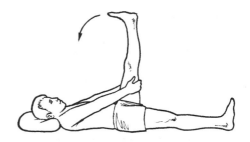

Calf stretch (gastrocnemius)
Stand with affected leg back in a walking position
Lean forwards (can use chair/wall for support)
Keep the back leg straight, heel on ground
Feel the stretch in calf
Hold for 20 seconds, repeat 5 times

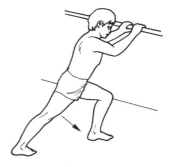

Postoperative management and advice

Total knee replacement (TKR)

Patients are advised not to kneel directly on their knee replacement (for the future – unless absolutely necessary). However, apart from this, there are no specific contraindications in terms of what patients can or cannot do following this operation. They will have rehabilitation whilst an inpatient and will be discharged when assessed as functionally able. The patient will have a home exercise programme to continue with and outpatient physiotherapy is organized if deemed necessary. Patients appear to have to work harder to regain range of movement following TKR in comparison to hip replacements and the range of movement obtained varies. The aim is to obtain 90 degrees of knee flexion postoperatively (70 degrees minimum). Patients will normally have walking aids (crutches or sticks) which they can gradually discard as they feel able. If knee movement is progressively decreasing or patients are having increasing difficulty with activities of daily living, referral for therapy is indicated. Signs of inflammation should be heeded with reduced activity, ice and medication.

Arthroscopy

Diagnostic arthroscopy washouts: These procedures may result in pain and swelling which may take up to 2 weeks to settle. Patients are normally seen by a physiotherapist and advised on a home exercise programme. Outpatient physiotherapy may be arranged, depending on the pathology found and the level of disability the patient is experiencing.

Arthroscopy meniscectomy: These patients may follow a similar routine to above unless they have a meniscus **repair**, where weightbearing may be restricted for up to 6 weeks.

Anterior cruciate ligament reconstruction

Numerous postoperative regimes are used, therefore check local protocols. These can vary from immobilization in casts for 6 weeks to immediate mobilization and weightbearing as tolerated. Comprehensive rehabilitation is normally instigated via the hospital orthopaedic or physiotherapy department and may continue for 6 months.

Examples of return to functional activities for those with immediate mobilization and a weightbearing programme following reconstruction, using the middle third of the patellar tendon, are approximately: sedentary work – 3–4 weeks; driving – 4–6 weeks; manual work – 8 weeks.

Foot and ankle

General advice for people with foot and ankle problems

- With recent onset ankle injuries advise rest in elevation with ice and compression. Address problems with gait (see next point). If not improving (within days), refer to a chartered physiotherapist.
- If unable to weightbear comfortably, and there is a significantly altered gait pattern, use sticks and crutches to aim to normalize the gait pattern. Use stick in **opposite** hand to side with the problem.
- Encourage movement without loading or twisting stresses (i.e. non-weightbearing exercises, progress to exercises in sitting and then to standing).
- Try 'contrast baths' – using alternate hot and cold immersions for pain relief (30 seconds to 1 minute in each for up to 10 minutes).
- Wear good supportive and appropriate footwear (particularly if partaking in running/sports). Be aware that high heel tabs can aggravate (or cause) some Achilles tendonitis problems. If necessary advise patients to cut the heel tabs down.

- Do not return to running or sports involving running unless patient can go up onto tiptoe on symptomatic side and hop on that leg without symptoms. In addition, change in direction at speed may be needed, therefore figure of 8 running with direction changes, etc. should be practised and a general training warm up before returning to their sport.

Ankle exercises

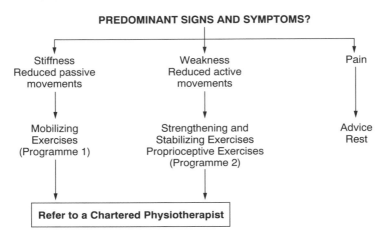

PREDOMINANT SIGNS AND SYMPTOMS?

Stiffness Reduced passive movements	Weakness Reduced active movements	Pain
Mobilizing Exercises (Programme 1)	Strengthening and Stabilizing Exercises Proprioceptive Exercises (Programme 2)	Advice Rest

Refer to a Chartered Physiotherapist

Foot exercises

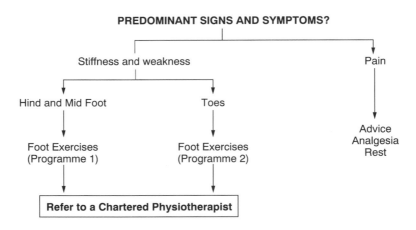

PREDOMINANT SIGNS AND SYMPTOMS?

Stiffness and weakness — Pain

Hind and Mid Foot	Toes
Foot Exercises (Programme 1)	Foot Exercises (Programme 2)

Advice Analgesia Rest

Refer to a Chartered Physiotherapist

Ankle mobilizing exercises

Ankle Programme 1

For patients with predominant signs and symptoms of **ankle stiffness**.

Start weightbearing exercises as soon as possible as they are more functionally relevant.

Non-weightbearing exercises
Ankle plantarflexion
Sit with leg supported (in elevation if swelling present)
Heel off end of bed/pillow
Point toes and foot down
Repeat 10 times

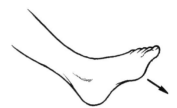

Ankle dorsiflexion
Sit with leg supported (in elevation if swelling present)
Heel off end of bed/pillow
Pull toes up towards knee
Use a scarf/belt to give extra pressure
Repeat 10 times

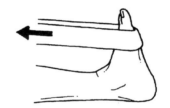

Ankle inversion and eversion
Sit with leg supported (in elevation if swelling present)
Heel off end of bed/pillow
Turn soles of feet:
(i)   to face each other
(ii)   away from each other
Keep knees/legs still
Repeat 10 times each movement

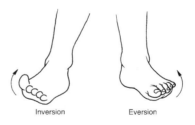

Inversion   Eversion

Progress to

Ankle plantarflexion and dorsiflexion in sitting
Sitting with feet on floor
Raise heels
Then raise toes
Alternate feet (like walking pattern)
Repeat 10 times each direction

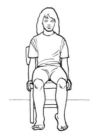

Weightbearing exercises
Ankle dorsiflexion – calf stretches
Stand with affected leg back in a walking position
Lean forwards (can use chair/wall for support)
Keep the back leg straight, heel on ground
Feel the stretch in calf
Hold 20 seconds, repeat 5 times

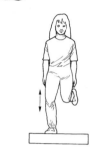

Ankle dorsiflexion – small dips
Stand sideways on a step/large book
Keep foot flat
Bend knee (so it is moving over second toe)
Hold on for balance if necessary (to begin with)
Repeat 10 times
Progress by standing facing forwards

Ankle plantorflexion – kneeling
Kneel on all fours
Gently sit back towards heels
Repeat 5–10 times

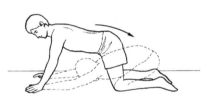

Ankle strengthening and stabilizing exercises

Ankle Programme 2

For patients with signs and symptoms of **ankle weakness and feelings of instability**. The muscles that commonly require strengthening are the ankle evertors and plantarflexors. Proprioceptive retraining is also important.

Ankle evertors
Sitting with foot dangling
Lift foot up with sole of foot facing outwards
Do not let knee move
Then lower it down slowly
Repeat 20–30 times
Progress by:
(i)   placing a weight on foot
(ii)   use elastic cord/rubber banding
(iii) can use other foot as resistance (cross feet)

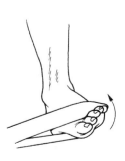

Ankle plantarflexors

Standing on both legs, weight equal on both feet
Go up onto tiptoe
Rest down
Try and make symptomatic side work at least 50%
Repeat 20 times
Progress by:
(i)   when on tiptoe, step to the side with other leg
(ii)   tiptoe walk
(iii)   do exercise standing on one leg
(iv)   start with heel over the side of step to get stretch
(v)   hop

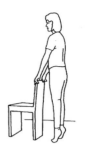

Static balance

Try and stand on one leg
Eyes open, eyes closed
Progress by repeating but on tiptoe

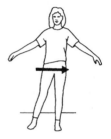

Dynamic balance

Stand on one leg
Keep body upright
Bend knee slowly, making sure knee is moving over second toe
Keep heel on the ground
Start with small dips and increase gradually (without pain)
Repeat 10–15 times, once a day minimum
Progress by:
(i)   hopping side to side (keeping alignment)
(ii)   Hopping forwards and back (keeping alignment)

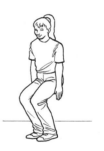

Foot exercises

Foot Programme 1

For patients with signs and symptoms relating to the **hind and mid foot**.

Intrinsics

Sit with foot on floor
Keep toes straight
Draw foot up as if it has become 'shortened'
Hold for 5 seconds
Repeat 20 times
(Can do this with shoes on, and in standing)

Calf stretches
Stand with affected leg back in a walking
position
Lean forwards (can use chair/wall for
support)
Keep the back leg straight, heel on
ground
Feel the stretch in calf
Hold for 20 seconds, repeat 5 times

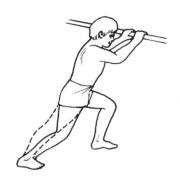

Repeat with same position as above, but
bend the back leg
Keep heel on ground
Feel stretch in calf, possibly nearer
Achilles tendon
Hold for 20 seconds, repeat 5 times

Tiptoe standing
Push up onto toes
Lower slowly
Progress to do without support (balance
or some weight)
Then progress to do on one leg
Repeat 20 times

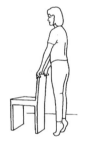

Dynamic alignment work in standing
Stand with feet hip width apart
Keep body upright
Bend knees fairly slowly, making sure
knees are moving over second toe. When
looking down inside knees, big toes
should be seen
Keep heels on the ground
Start with small dips and increase
gradually (without pain)
Repeat 10–15 times, once a day minimum
Progress further by doing on one leg,
maintaining balance

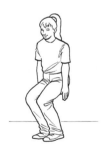

Foot exercises

Foot Programme 2

For patients with signs and symptoms in the **forefoot (toes)**.

Toe flexion

Sit with a strip of paper towel
or a thin towel under foot
Curl toes up to crumple towel
under foot
Repeat 10 times

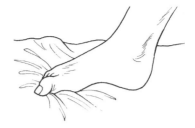

Toe extension

Sit with foot flat on ground
Raise heel, keeping toes on the
ground
Get bend at metatarso-
phalangeal joint
Repeat 5–10 times

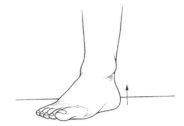

Toe abduction

This is difficult to do but does
improve with practice
Sit with foot on ground
Spread toes apart and together
Try and take big toe out to
side (towards the other foot)
Repeat 5–10 times (or until
fatigued)

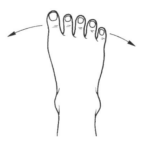

Postoperative management and advice

Patients are advised to:

- Elevate the foot/feet until the wounds are healed.
- Try and wear spacious and supportive footwear. Gradually build up their tolerance to wearing shoes again, starting with a few minutes each day.

Bunion surgery (bunionectomy, Kellers, Mitchell's osteotomy)

Patients are normally mobilized, heel-walking with crutches after 48 hours bed rest. They are discharged when safe for functional requirements, usually 2–3 days postoperatively.

Plaster of Paris or splints are maintained for 8 weeks. During this time patients gradually increase their walking ability, discarding walking aids as able. It may be a further 8 weeks until a shoe can be worn at all, and 6 months for full recovery.

No specific physiotherapy or exercise programme is implemented.

Fusion of toes

The fusion may be held by a pin for 6–8 weeks. This is removed in the outpatient clinic. The postoperative management is similar in format to bunion surgery (see above).

Achilles tendon rupture

Management of this varies (conservative versus surgical repair and early mobilization versus cast immobilization in both cases). Rehabilitation will normally be instigated according to local instructions. Patients normally need help to regain propulsive and proprioceptive function of the lower limb.

Appendix 11.1

Heat

Heat is used for pain relief, reducing muscle spasm, and increasing joint and/or soft tissue extensibility. It can also encourage the healing of injuries or in mild or chronic inflammation.

It can be given satisfactorily using

- hot water bottle;
- warm shower;
- warm bath;
- soaking hands/feet in warm water – using rubber gloves on hands will enable warmer water to be used for this area, without giving skin discomfort;
- warm swimming pool, jacuzzi;
- electrical heat pads.

The old fashioned infrared lamp is now rarely used and not recommended.

Heat should not be used on:

- acutely inflamed areas, e.g. hot joints, skin which has had radiotherapy or chemical irritants, acute dermatitis or eczema;
- areas with an absence of or poor thermal sensation;
- areas with ischaemia, which may not allow an adequate vasodilatory response (e.g. ateriosclerosis, Buerger's disease).

Patients with cardiovascular deficiencies or problems with heat-regulating mechanisms may be at risk if totally immersed in warm water.

Contrast baths

This involves immersion in alternate hot (40–45°C) and cold (from tap) water baths. It is useful for limb extremity problems. The limb part is first immersed in the hot bath for 3–4 minutes, and then placed in the cold bath for 1 minute. This cycle is repeated three or four times so that the process may last 15–20 minutes.

Cold

Cold is used for reducing pain and muscle spasm. It gives a strong sensory input which can give effective pain relief. It is beneficial in recent trauma in reducing bleeding and rate of swelling.

It can be applied in various different ways:

- **Ice pack:** Crushed ice or frozen peas (small particles make it more malleable) can be made into a pack. The ice can be wrapped in a wet towel and placed on a piece of paper towel over the skin. This does result in a wet mess, but it is effective in delivering cold to the tissues! If the ice or peas are wrapped or contained in plastic, a damp towel should be placed over the skin. This precaution reduces the risk of an ice burn (a thin layer of oil on the skin will also reduce this risk). In addition, advise the patients not to rest the weight of their body or body part on an ice pack (e.g. lying with leg resting on an ice pack under the calf).
- **Ice massage:** Using an ice cube or an ice 'lollipop'. The lollipop is made from water placed in a plastic cup with a stick in it and put in the freezer. The ice blocks are initially wetted and then rubbed over the painful areas in slow circular movements. The patient feels cold, burning to aching, and then a numbness which may take 5–10 minutes to achieve.
- **Ice baths:** This uses a mixture of flaked ice and cold tap water in a container or sink. The limb extremities can be placed into the iced water. The temperature can be changed by altering the proportions of ice to water. Temperatures of about 16–18°C can usually be tolerated for up to 20 minutes.
- **Ice towels:** This involves dipping a terry-towel into a mixture of crushed ice and water, then wringing it out and then wrapping it around the problem area for 2–3 minutes before replacing it with a new towel. This tends to be comfortable and does allow the patient to move with the towel on, but one gets very cold hands!
- **Commercially available cold packs (kept in the freezer):** These still should be applied with a wet towel over the skin. They are convenient but may not be as effective in delivering cold to the tissues.

There is the danger of tissue injury – an ice 'burn'. This can occasionally be seen on normal tissues as tenderness and an erythema of the skin, which can appear several hours after the application of ice. In more severe forms, there is fatty necrosis and bruising can accompany the above symptoms and may last for up to 3 weeks.

Caution is advised in the application of ice on areas with local autonomic pain or temperature disturbances.

Ice therapy may not be suitable for patients with medical conditions which will increase cold sensitivity, such as Raynaud's phenomenon, Buerger's diseases, cryoglobinaemia and cold urticaria.

Care should be taken when cooling large areas of the body in patients with hypertension and cardiac disease.

Appendix 11.2

Boots The Chemist have produced a catalogue, 'Active and Independent', price £1.00 if purchased.

The catalogue is comprehensive and includes aids and appliances for all aspects of daily living (kitchen, house, bathroom, bedroom and being 'out and about'). It has been compiled using expertise from the Chartered Society of Physiotherapy, the College of Occupational Therapsits, the Disabled Living Foundation and the Disabled Living Centres Council. It shows items that can be obtained and delivered to a patient's home (without extra cost) if the items are not held in stock.

If patients wish to purchase such appliances, this may be the easiest way in which to do so, or they can contact their local occupational therapy services (community or hospital, depending on the nature of their problem and recent management).

Further reading

Basmajian, J. V. and Wolf, S. L. (1990). *Therapeutic Exercise*, 5th edn. Williams and Wilkins, Baltimore.

Clinical Standards Advisory Group (1994). *Back Pain*, HMSO, London.

Jones, K. and Barker K. (1996). *Human Movement Explained*. Butterworth-Heinemann, Oxford.

Low J. and Reed, A. (1990). *Electrotherapy Explained*. Butterworth-Heinemann, Oxford.

Maitland, G. D. (1986). *Vertebral Manipulation*. 5th edn. Butterworth-Heinemann, Oxford.

McKenzie, R. (1983). *Treat Your Own Neck*. Spinal Publications, New Zealand.

McKenzie R. (1985). *Treat Your Own Back*. Spinal Publications, New Zealand.

Roland, M. and Dixon, M. (1989). The role of an educational booklet in managing patients presenting with back pain in primary care. In *Back Pain. New approaches to education and rehabilitation* (M. Roland and J. Jenner eds). Manchester University press, Manchester, pp. 84–92.

Index

[Pages with figures are marked by italic type; pages with tables are bold type]